The Placebo Effect

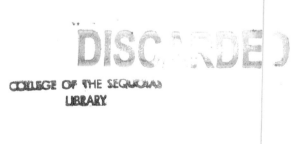

The Placebo Effect

An Interdisciplinary Exploration

Editor

Anne Harrington

Harvard University Press

Cambridge, Massachusetts
London, England

Copyright © 1997 by the President and Fellows of Harvard College
Printed in the United States of America

Third printing, 2000

First Harvard University Press paperback edition, 1999

Library of Congress Cataloging-in-Publication Data
The placebo effect : an interdisciplinary exploration / editor, Anne Harrington.
    p.   cm.
Includes bibliographical references and index.
ISBN 0-674-66984-3 (cloth)
ISBN 0-674-66986-X (pbk.)
1. Placebo (Medicine)—Congresses. I. Harrington, Anne, 1960– .
[DNLM: 1. Placebo effect—congresses.
2. Drug therapy—congresses.
3. Philosophy, Medical—congresses.
WB 330 P6965 1997]
RM331.P53 1997
615.5—dc21
DNLM/DLC
for Library of Congress   97-4324

This book is dedicated to the late Arthur Shapiro, M.D.,
in appreciation for his forty years of pioneering work
on the placebo effect.

Acknowledgments

This book is based on materials that were first presented at a three-day conference entitled "Placebo: Probing the Self-Healing Brain," held at Harvard University, December 7–10, 1994. That event was sponsored by the Harvard Mind, Brain, Behavior Initiative, an interfaculty venture at the university piloting new strategies in interdisciplinary dialogue, research, and teaching. The conceptual "making" of the meeting itself was an intense team effort by one of the "working groups" within the initiative, which was composed of Harvard faculty: John Dowling, Gordon Kaufman, Stephen Kosslyn, Elaine Scarry, Alan Stone, Lawrence Sullivan, and myself. I am grateful to the initiative for its faith in this venture. I also feel particularly indebted to its administrative director, Shawn Bohen, and her assistant, Christine Thurmond, for their unfailing, graceful, and practical support in putting together all the pieces of the actual event.

The initial inspiration for both the workshop and this volume came from conversations and work pursued within the MacArthur Foundation Research Network on Mind-Body Interactions. The network provided funding for an extensive literature review of placebo effects that has fundamentally shaped both the basic "argument" and the organization of this book. I thank my colleagues in the network for their engagement with me on these issues, especially Robert Rose and Kenneth Hugdahl, who traveled from far-flung places to participate in the conference itself.

My assistant, Billie Jo Joy, took on the arduous task of bringing all the material in this book into consistent format, ensuring readability and seeing that every correction and query was followed up and resolved. Her extraordinary initiative, intelligence, and focused care in this task have earned my deepest respect.

Contents

Introduction   1
    Anne Harrington

1 The Placebo: Is It Much Ado about Nothing?   12
    Arthur K. Shapiro and Elaine Shapiro

2 Clinical Reflections on the Placebo Phenomenon   37
    Howard Spiro

3 The Nocebo Phenomenon: Scope and Foundations   56
    Robert A. Hahn

4 The Doctor as Therapeutic Agent:
A Placebo Effect Research Agenda   77
    Howard Brody

5 Toward a Neurobiology of Placebo Analgesia   93
    Howard L. Fields and Donald D. Price

6 The Contribution of Desire and Expectation to Placebo
Analgesia: Implications for New Research Strategies   117
    Donald D. Price and Howard L. Fields

7 The Role of Conditioning in Pharmacotherapy   138
        Robert Ader

8 Specifying Nonspecifics: Psychological Mechanisms
      of Placebo Effects   166
        Irving Kirsch

9 Placebo, Pain, and Belief: A Biocultural Model   187
        David B. Morris

     Placebo: Conversations at the Disciplinary Borders   208
        Edited by Anne Harrington

     Contributors   251

     Index   254

The Placebo Effect

Introduction

Anne Harrington

In the clinic, it has been long acknowledged that "sham" treatments like sugar pills or injections with saline solution have the capacity to rally healing processes, sometimes of a dramatic nature, within patients. This acknowledgment, however, has as often as not been marked by ambivalence and distaste. The very word we use to name the phenomenon at hand, "placebo response," speaks to our ambivalence. *Placebo* is Latin for "I shall please" (and the opening phrase of the Catholic vespers for the dead, from which the medical term, ironically enough, derived). Placebos are therefore typically defined as sham treatments (bread pills, inert tonics, and so on) that physicians dole out merely to "please" or placate anxious or insatiable patients. And even when these physicians are convinced that impressive forces may be rallied through their maneuvers, they often cannot shake themselves free of the conviction that this practice is at best unreal and at worst chicanery.

The problems raised for medicine by placebo phenomena, however, are not only ethical: they are also epistemological. Placebos are the ghosts that haunt our house of biomedical objectivity, the creatures that rise up from the dark and expose the paradoxes and fissures in our own self-created definitions of the real and active factors in treatment. On the one hand, we acknowledge the power and ubiquity of placebo responses by our requirement that all new drugs be tested in double-blind placebo-controlled situations; however, we then define those same responses as the "non-specific noise" in the treatment to be

1

subtracted out of the picture. We often fail to notice that these factors are not *inherently* nonspecific but are only so because insufficient energy and attention has been spent on specifying them.

In 1969, the social psychologist W. J. McGuire described "three stages in the life of an artifact": first it is ignored; then it is controlled for its presumed contaminating effects; and, finally, it is studied as an important phenomenon in its own right. Currently placebo effects are still more often controlled away than studied, but one can track a thin trajectory of research literature that, from the 1950s up to our own time, has also attempted to make the case for investigating these effects in their own right. Tracking these literatures as they have developed across time is an interesting exercise, not only because of the different kinds of information that each perspective brings to an elucidation of the phenomenon at hand, but also because each represents a distinct answer to the question of what the task of explaining placebo effects should look like. In fact, we do not just go out and investigate the placebo phenomenon: we also constantly make decisions about *what* we think is important to know about it and what kinds of explanations we are prepared to consider to be illuminating and rigorous.

Early clinical articles like Henry Beecher's "The Powerful Placebo" (1955) had made it clear that placebos could cause objective (structurally and functionally measurable) changes in physiological functioning, some of which (as researchers of the time marveled) could even "exceed those attributable to potent pharmacologic action." Nevertheless, even researchers who emphasized the physiological potency of placebos still seemed to suggest that explanations for that potency needed to be sought within some free-floating Cartesian room (often decked out with quasi-Freudian furniture) that possessed no clear means of "talking" with the body that it was influencing in such useful ways. In a sense, the original decision to define *placebo* as the imaginary term in medicine's algebraic formula of treatment may have forced people's hands here: if an intervention that has been defined as unreal or inert turns out to work through biochemical or physiological mediators, then how could one continue to consider the intervention merely a placebo?

Most of the early psychological explanations tended in the first instance to focus on the patient. It was clear that not everyone responded to placebos (a widely cited statistic, going back to Henry Beecher's 1955 study held that 30–40 percent of any treated group responded to placebo; the figure was believed to be somewhat higher—about 55 percent—for pain relief). What kind of personality structure, then, responded to imaginary medications? Often there was a quasi-pathological thrust to the attempts to answer this question, a vague undertone of condescension consistent with the general ambivalence that most physicians felt towards placebos in general, and perhaps especially towards the patients who could be fooled by them. Using various standardized psychological tests and psychodynamic profiles, researchers thus explored the extent to which so-called "placebo reactors" might be unusually suggestible (or, alternatively, unusually hypnotizable); might have unstable reality-testing skills, might suffer from repression, hysterical tendencies, or other neurotic symptoms; might exhibit unusual compliant, submissive personality traits; or might even be less intelligent overall than nonplacebo responders (see, for example, Lasagna et al. 1954; for a recent study in this tradition, see Reich 1990).

By the 1970s, however, there was a growing consensus that no consistent "placebo responder" was out there to be found, and such books as Jerome Frank's masterly 1973 *Persuasion and Healing* (Frank 1973) began to emphasize the greater importance of immediate situational and interpersonal factors. Depending on the quality of the doctor-patient relationship, the nature of the "socially defined symbols of healing" that are used, or any number of other conditions, the same individual might be responsive to placebos or not. As early as the 1960s writers like Arthur Shapiro had reminded people that the physician was also important in the dyadic dance of healing, and proposed that doctors—independent of what they did—were actually potent placebos in their own right (Shapiro 1969). He and others enumerated a number of specific variables that might endow some physicians with particular curative mana: enthusiasm for treatment, apparent warm feelings for the patient, confidence, and authority. Some who gave this exercise an explicit psychoanalytic spin proposed that the physician in a placebo-treatment situation acted as a parental transference figure onto whom vulnerable patients projected childlike feelings of trust and submission along with expectations of being "made better" (discussed, for example, in Byerly 1976).

Others in these years began to dispute the substance behind some of the more fervent evangelical reports of miracle placebo cures and scoffed that placebo effects actually did not involve real change in a patient's physical state at all. Instead, they maintained, the placebo effects simply represented a *misattribution* by the patient of various naturally occurring and ambiguous changes in his or her clinical condition (Gibbons and Hormuth 1981; Ross and Olson 1981). Motivated to believe that he or she is being helped and wanting to please the physician, a patient will tend to downplay or censor his or her awareness of negative changes and will give undue weight to positive changes. He or she may then selectively attribute all welcomed alterations to the placebo drug. In a variation on this argument, others agreed that placebos did not change the supposed nonnegotiable *physiological* realities inherent to a particular medical condition. However, they proposed that placebo might ameliorate the distressing *subjective* concomitants of somatic illness, such as anxiety. (The subjective experience of pain, for example, is known to be intensified by anxiety; see Spiro (Chapter 2) for a tempered defense of this position.)

Then, in the late 1970s, two things happened in the brain sciences that seemed to raise the stakes considerably on the placebo question. The first of these was an outgrowth of the much-heralded discovery of certain naturally occurring substances in the brain called endorphins. Chemically similar to opium-derived narcotics, endorphins attach themselves to the same receptor sites in the brain as morphine and thus appear to be the brain's own natural painkillers. In 1978, Jon D. Levine, N. C. Gordon, and Howard L. Fields reported evidence that at least some forms of placebo analgesia were mediated by these same endogenous opioids (Levine, Gordon, and Fields 1978). These researchers had found that when patients receiving placebo medication for postoperative pain were given naloxone, a substance that blocks opiate receptors, the effects of placebo were inhibited.

Lively controversy ensued over both the meaning and the consistency of the findings, especially when several other studies showed that naloxone could increase postoperative pain independently of placebo (see, for example, Gracely et al. 1983). In addition, it was pointed out that the data on endorphins spoke only to the rather limited question of placebo *analgesia* and had nothing to say about the many other kinds of documented effects that had been associated with placebo interventions (a point discussed in Kirsch 1990). And finally there were questions about just what kind of finding the endorphin-placebo link really was: even if endorphins did mediate some kinds of placebo analgesia, that analgesia was not thereby explained (as some seemed to imply). Endorphin release, rather, became just one more placebo-generated phenomenon to be explained—and we still did not understand the processes whereby a person's belief in a sham treatment could send a message to his or her pituitary gland to release its own endogenous pharmaceutics (see Chapters 5 and 6).

Nevertheless, the discovery that endorphins might be involved in at least some forms of placebo analgesia (and the basic claim has held up) seemed so exciting on its own terms that there was a tendency to be relatively undeterred by the caveats and cautions of the gadflies. In fact, the intensity of the reaction within the scientific community suggests that the placebo-endorphin link came to mean something more than itself. It acted, not just as a set of findings, but as a notice to the hardheaded, physiologically oriented members of the biomedical community that there was work to be done in this realm after all. Placebo, an "imaginary" treatment, had been found to have some solid flesh on its bones after all.

The second event that raised the biomedical stakes on the placebo question came in 1975. In this year, Robert Ader and his coworkers reported the results of a study with rats that involved a pairing (initially unintentional) of saccharin-flavored drinking water with injections of cyclophosphamide, an immunosuppressive and nausea-inducing drug (Ader and Cohen 1975). At this time, the immune system was believed to be a self-contained system not susceptible to influences from the central nervous system. Yet, when a subgroup of mice who were not given further injections continued to be fed drinks of saccharin water, they kept dying at high rates. It seemed that the saccharin drink, because it was originally associated by the rats with the injections, now triggered the same immunosuppressive effects as the cyclophosphamide itself. By "teaching" the rats to associate the saccharin water with the agency of the active substance, Ader had induced the immune systems of rats to behave in ways different from normal. In this sense, he had created an experimental placebo whose effects on physiological functioning were incontrovertible. The fact that he had achieved this in rats rather than in humans was a further blockbuster, because it undermined the frequent assumption that placebo effects were a product of peculiarly human interpersonal processes and unconscious wishes.

Actually, some researchers since the 1950s had tried to make the case that placebo effects were just a consequence of classical conditioning (or, in some formulations, of nonconscious associative learning processes). Just as Pavlov's dogs were conditioned to respond to an irrelevant stimulus (a bell) as if it were meat powder, so individuals who have had successful trials with active medications (the unconditioned stimulus) become conditioned to respond to inert symbols of medicine (the conditioned stimulus) *as if* they were also active (Gliedman et al. 1956; Herrnstein 1962). The original conditioning model of placebo effects, however, had not found a great deal of resonance within the psychoanalytically oriented world of mental medicine; now Ader's work, with its startling apparent implications for health, helped put conditioning theory back on the front page of promising strategies for cracking open the secrets of this phenomenon.

Very soon, however, other voices continued to insist on the insufficiency of the conditioning paradigm and to argue that the last word had not yet been said about the peculiarly human face of the placebo story. Social psychologist Irving Kirsch, for example, stressed that placebo-generated effects often followed a "logic of expectation" that was different from what would be expected if placebos merely evoked a conditioned reaction to some corresponding active agent (Kirsch 1985). The experiences of people who drink placebo alcohol are more closely linked to their culture's understanding of what it means to be "under the influence" than they are to the actual pharmacological action of real alcohol. In addition, there was evidence in the literature that the imagined effects of a substance can sometimes directly countermand its actual pharmacology. Back in 1950, Stewart Wolf reported giving ipecac (an emetic) to a severely nauseous pregnant woman and vigorously assuring her that this was medication that would help her; a balloon in her stomach showed that her stomach began contracting normally within minutes after "treatment" (Wolf 1950).

To add a final layer of complication to the debates, a cadre of medical anthropologists like Arthur Kleinman, Robert Hahn, and

David Moerman began in the 1980s to argue that nothing less than a broad sociocultural framework would do for making sense of the questions raised by placebo effects. They envisioned placebo as a form of ritualized healing through symbols, comparable to the healing rituals practiced in societies across the world (practices that these societies in no sense consider to be imaginary or sham, whatever the opinions of the Western world). The anthropologists asserted that symbolic healing of other cultures is often quite effective, just as placebos are often effective, and that they are so because human beings structure and partly create their experiences of illness and recovery through shared symbols and metaphors (Moerman 1983; Hahn and Kleinman 1983). In short, said the anthropologists, placebos were symbols of healing, but symbols have real effects on human bodies. Failing to understand this fact had blinded Western high-tech medicine to ways in which it still shared key formal properties with the bone-pointing or charismatic religious healing practices of groups that Western scientists and physicians too often did not understand, let alone appreciate.

We enter the 1990s, in short, with a range of diverse, disciplinary perspectives on the placebo effect that jostle for a hearing, and at the moment we know of no higher formula for either adjudicating between or synthesizing them. A decade ago, White, Tursky, and Schwartz (1985) published a volume that brought together the most important disciplinary perspectives on the placebo. At the end of the volume, the editors reviewed the contributions and called for an "integrative synthesis of all relevant views and factors" (a dizzying list). Their exhortation, however, was ultimately too daunting and nonspecific to function as a prod for much, if any, renewed interdisciplinary effort among the relevant parties. What seems clearer today is that interdisciplinarity is not readily achieved just by giving "air time" to different points of view (valuable as that is). There are methodological, epistemological, even metaphysical tensions involved in the attempt to arrive at an understanding greater than the sum of its parts; and these tensions are not readily resolved, even by invoking concepts of "levels and systems."

The tensions are especially great when one attempts to move between the divide that separates the explanatory strategies of the so-called cultural or hermeneutic sciences (roughly concerned with "meaning") and the so-called natural sciences (roughly committed to explanations in terms of "mechanism"). Because placebos as a phenomenon seem to hover ambiguously at the crossroads between these two perspectives, they are at once a frustration and a wonderful challenge. Whatever additional role placebos play in the worlds of medical science, they certainly function as a powerful reminder to thoughtful scholars and researchers that our minds, brains, and bodies navigate a far more seamless reality than we, in our insular academic departments, know how to study.

Placebos, in other words, are not only puzzles to be "solved," but—to the extent that they *elude* ready solutions—they also teach us how far we still are from closure on the question of what it will mean to create a science subtle and complex enough to encompass all that is entailed in being human. This is the view of placebos, at any rate, that has animated the orientation and substance of the present volume. This volume had its origins in an interdisciplinary conference that convened at Harvard University for three days in December 1994 under the sponsorship of the Harvard Mind, Brain, Behavior Interfaculty Initiative (with initial research support from the MacArthur Research Network on Mind-Body Interactions). The goal of that gathering had been to push the envelope of thinking on placebo in ways that might help reshape how the problem is conceived and studied. Scholars and scientists with expertise ranging from religious studies to molecular biology came together to ponder how to do better justice to the integrated ways in which sociocultural meanings and physiological mechanisms function fluidly within a single human being.

The results of our efforts are documented in this volume. The book opens with a summative paper by the late Arthur Shapiro, whose career in placebo research stretches back almost forty years, and his wife and colleague, Elaine Shapiro. The Shapiros provide an authoritative historical review of the place of placebos in the history of medicine; ask why interest in them is currently as pronounced as it is; and undertake a sharp-eyed analysis of the methodological difficulties involved in really nailing down scientifically just what placebos can and cannot do. Howard Spiro supplies a clinician's perspective on placebo effects; he is concerned less with the science of placebos and more with their functioning in the real world of pain, suffering, care, and healing. He asks as many questions about what placebos mean to doctors and their therapeutic tasks as he does about what they mean for patients and their treatment.

Howard L. Fields, who in the 1970s helped discover that placebos given to relieve pain can stimulate release of endogenous opiates, teams up in this volume with Donald Price to suggest that new advances in knowledge suggest that we can now integrate those earlier findings within a more comprehensive model of psychoneurophysiological pain modulation. The second coauthored paper by this team (with Donald D. Price as first author) elaborates on the foundations set down by the first paper, by identifying what the authors believe to be the key psychological mechanisms operative in placebo responsivity. They propose that these mechanisms can be operationalized and studied, with the goal ultimately of integrating our understanding of them with neurophysiological levels of explanation.

Robert Ader, whose work on immune system conditioning helped launch the field of psychoneuroimmunology, contributes here an elegant and data-dense defense of placebo as a conditioned response. Ader has some particular points to make about how a better understanding of placebo action should alter our understanding of what happens and is required in pharmacotherapeutic regimens. Irving Kirsch reviews the literature on psychological mechanisms of placebo effects, focusing particularly on evidence that, although conditioning explanations can take us some way towards an explanation of placebos, they cannot take us the whole distance. He proposes instead that placebos be understood as direct effects of individual "expectancies."

Robert A. Hahn helps us at once to bend and enlarge our understanding of the terrain in which we are walking with a paper, not on placebos, but on so-called "nocebos"—imagined, expected, or symbolic practices or interventions that cause distress, sickness, or even death (the phenomenon once called "voodoo death"). Hahn differentiates these from placebos, while arguing that nevertheless they share with placebos the quality of being "culturogenic"—products of culturally derived expectations that interact directly with individual physiology. Howard Brody focuses on placebos as products of narrative and meaning-making, which he sees as interpersonal effects of the doctor-patient relationship. Brody then imagines what it might be like to integrate a meaning-oriented approach to placebo with an appropriately subtle and sophisticated neurophysiology that could explain why meaningful stimuli have a healing effect. David B. Morris moves in a somewhat similar direction as Brody. Building on arguments developed in detail in his earlier work on the "culture of pain," he argues that placebos have irreducible qualities that demand what he calls a biocultural approach to their elucidation. As he puts it, "humans activate the neurobiological circuits required for placebo effects through the subtle and diffuse experience of living within the inescapably meaning-rich domain of culture."

The final part of this book shares highlights from a rather extraordinary dialogue that took place over three days between the diverse group of scholars at the 1994 Harvard meeting. Although we were there to discuss placebo effects, we were continually inspired to redraw the problem at hand in ever more generous strokes. Our conversations roamed over themes as varied as why people "wait" until holidays to get ill; what is the "will to live"; what is the therapeutic power that lies in telling one's "story"; what are the limits of scientific explanation; what it means to know; why consciousness matters; what healing by "faith" might entail; whether one can "die of fear"; why placebos shame science as much as interest it; and more. As we spoke, we also all began to move beyond mere irritation at not having our views immediately understood and to find intellectual intrigue in our differences. We did not end our three days of intensive exchange with a clear strategy about what now needs to be done to understand how the cultural and symbolic become embodied or how the bodily and physiological become acculturated. We did not even achieve consensus that this was the obvious, desirable goal. By and large, however, we were able to agree that the liminal reality of placebo effects—existing somewhere between meaning and mechanism—did offer disciplinary research and scholarship rich opportunities to stretch in ways that promised to leave none of the parties involved in the undertaking unchanged.

References

Ader, R. A., and N. Cohen. 1975. "Behaviorally Conditioned Immunosuppression." *Psychosomatic Medicine*, 37:333–340.

Byerly, H. 1976. "Explaining and Exploiting Placebo Effects." *Perspectives in Biology and Medicine,* 19:423–436.

Frank, Jerome D. 1973. *Persuasion and Healing* (rev. ed.). Baltimore: Johns Hopkins University Press.

Gibbons, F., and S. E. Hormuth. 1981. "Motivational Factors in Placebo Responsivity." *Psychopharmacology Bulletin,* 17:77–79.

Gliedman, L. H., W. H. Gantt, and H. A. Teitelbaum. 1956. "Some Implications of Conditional Reflex Studies for Placebo Research." *American Journal of Psychiatry,* 113:1103–1107.

Gordon, N. C., and J. D. Levine. 1981. "Physiological Substrates of Placebo Analgesia." *Psychopharmacology Bulletin,* 17:76–77.

Gracely, R. H., R. Dubner, P. J. Wolskee, and W. R. Deeter. 1983. "Placebo and Naloxone Can Alter Post-surgical Pain by Separate Mechanisms." *Nature,* 306:264–265.

Hahn, Robert A., and Arthur Kleinman. 1983. "Belief as Pathogen, Belief as Medicine: 'Voodoo Death' and the 'Placebo Phenomenon' in Anthropological Perspective." *Medical Anthropology Quarterly,* 4:16–19.

Herrnstein, R. J. 1962. "Placebo Effect in the Rat." *Science,* 138:677–678.

Kirsch, I. 1985. "Response Expectancy as a Determinant of Experience and Behavior." *American Psychologist,* 40:1189–1202.

———. 1990. *Changing Expectations: A Key to Effective Psychotherapy.* Pacific Grove, Calif.: Brooks/Cole.

Lasagna, L., F. Mosteller, J. M. von Felsinger, and H. K. Beecher. 1954. "A Study of the Placebo Response." *American Journal of Medicine,* 16:770–779.

Levine, J. D., N. C. Gordon, and H. L. Fields. 1978. "The Mechanism of Placebo Analgesia." *Lancet,* 2:654–657.

Moerman, Daniel. 1983. "General Medical Effectiveness and Human Biology: Placebo Effects in the Treatment of Ulcer Disease." *Medical Anthropology Quarterly,* 14:3, 13–16.

Reich, J. 1990. "The Effect of Personality on Placebo Response in Panic Patients." *Journal of Nervous and Mental Diseases,* 178:699–702.

Ross, M., and J. M. Olson. 1981. "An Expectancy-attribution Model of the Effects of Placebos." *Psychological Review,* 88:408–437.

Shapiro, A. K. 1969. "Iatroplacebogenics." *International Pharmacopsychiatry,* 2:215–248.

Spiro, Howard M. 1986. *Doctors, Patients, and Placebos.* New Haven: Yale University Press.

White, L., B. Tursky, and G. E. Schwartz. 1985. *Placebo: Theory, Research, and Mechanisms.* New York: Guilford Press.

Wolf, Stewart. 1950. "Effects of Suggestion and Conditioning on the Action of Chemical Agents in Human Subjects—The Pharmacology of Placebos." *Journal of Clinical Investigation,* 29:100–109.

The Placebo:
Is It Much Ado about Nothing?

1

Arthur K. Shapiro
Elaine Shapiro

Is the placebo much ado about nothing? The answer is both NO because it has powerful therapeutic effects and YES because there are such faddish exaggerations about the extent of placebo power.

Definition of a Placebo

What is a placebo? The placebo would be unimportant if it included only intentional use of inert substances, such as Sacchari Lactis, because few healers intentionally use inert placebos. Many more healers use ineffective or placebo dosages. However, the most extensive use of placebos are the many treatments erroneously believed by both healers and patients to be effective.

Our definition, which is based on the etymology of the word itself, methodological principles, and heuristic considerations, is any therapy prescribed knowingly or unknowingly by a healer, or used by laymen, for its therapeutic effect on a symptom or disease, but which actually is ineffective or not specifically effective for the symptom or disorder being treated. We define the *placebo effect* as the nonspecific, psychological, or psychophysiologic therapeutic effect produced by a placebo, or the effect of spontaneous improvement attributed to the placebo (Shapiro 1968; *Oxford English Dictionary* 1989; Shapiro and Shapiro in prep).

Simply stated, a therapy may be used with the knowledge that it is a placebo or may be given in the belief that it is not a placebo, but by objective evaluation is a placebo. The placebo may be an inert sugar pill, an active drug, or any treatment no matter how potentially specific or by whom administered.

Placebo Effects in Prescientific Medicine

The panorama of treatment since antiquity provides ample support for the conviction that, until recently, the history of medical treatment is essentially the history of the placebo effect. Just consider the number of drugs that are known from antiquity (Garrison 1921; Majno 1975; Estes 1989; Shapiro and Shapiro in prep).

The Yellow Emperor Huang Ti mentions over 2,000 drugs and 16,000 prescriptions that were used in China for 2,500 years without major change. Sumerian-Babylonian-Assyrian records refer to 265 remedies. The Ebers Papyrus names 842 prescriptions and more than 700 drugs. Over 600 drugs were used in ancient India. The Hippocratic Corpus mentions 195 to 400 drugs. Galen's pharmacopoeia, which dominated treatment for 1,500 years and completely disappeared only at the onset of scientific medicine in the nineteenth century, totaled 820 placebo remedies. Despite this, Galen proclaimed, "Never as yet have I gone astray, whether in treatment or in prognosis, as have so many other physicians of great reputation. If anyone wishes to gain fame . . . all that he needs is to accept what I have been able to establish." Yet he had the insight to observe, "He cures most successfully in whom the people have the most confidence."

The astonishing total of these ancient remedies is about 4,785 drugs and 16,842 prescriptions. Even more startling is that with only a few possible but unlikely speculative exceptions, all were placebos. And these are limited to only the written records of drugs and prescriptions and do not include many others that were not recorded.

Moreover, similar extensive lists of placebo drugs could be compiled from all medical pharmacopoeias into the twentieth century. For example, the first three editions of the London Pharmacopoeia (Garrison 1921) published in the seventeenth century included such useless drugs as usnea (moss from the skull of victims of violent death), Vigo's plaster (viper's flesh, live frogs and worms), Gascoyne's powder (bezoar, amber, pearls, crabs' eyes, coral, and black tops of crabs' claws), triangular Wormian bone from the juncture of the sagittal and lambdoid sutures of the skull of an executed criminal, theriac, mattioli, mithridate, bile, blood, bee glue, bones, bone marrow, claws, cuttlefish, cock's comb, cast-off snake skin, fox lung, fat, fur, feathers, hair, horns, hoofs, isinglass, lozenges of dried viper, oil of brick, ants, and wolves, powder of precious stones, seasilk, sponge, scorpions, swallows' nest, spider webs, raw silk, teeth, viscera, worms, wood lice, human placenta and perspiration, saliva of a fasting man, sexual organs, and excreta of all sorts. Although pharmacopoeias continued to drop questionable remedies, in 1746 the London Pharmacopoeia retained mithridate, theriac, bezoars, crabs' eyes, and wood lice; and it included many new drugs which were no more effective than those that they replaced. This substitution of one placebo for another is reflected in the loosely paraphrased old adage, "Hurry, hurry, use the new drug before it stops healing."

Placebo Panaceas

Cure-alls were used extensively for centuries (Garrison 1921; Haggard 1933; Major 1954; Watson 1966; Majno 1975; Estes 1989). *Theriac,* medicine's universal panacea, and one of the oldest, most expensive, and long lasting, contained from 33 to over 100 substances and took months to years to concoct. Theriac's main ingredient was viper's flesh, medicine's magical restorative—since vipers shed and grow new skin— and theriac often contained opium for good measure. Galen wrote a whole book about it called *Theriake,* and theriac was included in the 1872 German and 1874 French pharmacopoeia. It could even be bought as Venice treacle in Vienna as late as World War II. *Mattioli,* the drug with the most ingredients, contained up to 230 substances. *Unicorn horn,* the most expensive remedy, sold for 10 times its weight in gold in the sixteenth century, equivalent to $500,000 today. *Bezoar stone,* a universal antidote believed to be the crystallized tear from the eye of a deer bitten by a snake, was actually gall stones or concretions found in the stomachs and intestines of animals such as the goat, and was often counterfeited with the substitution of pebbles. *Mandrake,* the drug most frequently cited by Shakespeare, was used by Babylonians, Hebrews, Greeks, Romans, and early twentieth-century physicians to treat almost every malady at one time or another. According to popular superstition, the mandrake, which resembled a man, would shriek when pulled from the earth. Because it was believed that a person hearing the shriek would go insane or die, a horn was blown to drown out the shriek. For further protection, a dog was tied to the plant with a rope and food left nearby. When the dog attempted to escape or reach the food, it pulled out the root, went mad, and died. *Powdered Egyptian mummy* was another expensive universal remedy, albeit one that could kill, if the real stuff were taken, because arsenic was the main ingredient in the embalming process. A more specific remedy was *stone cutting.* Physicians and stone-cutting quacks treated insanity, idiocy, and other mental disorders from the fifteenth to the seventeenth century by surreptitiously removing a palmed stone from a superficial scalp incision. This may be the origin of the common phrase "rocks in your head" to denote insanity.

Patients continued to submit to purging, puking, poisoning, cutting, cupping, blistering, bleeding, freezing, heating, sweating, leeching, and shocking. Despite the extensive use of these noxious methods and many other bizarre substances, physicians continued to be respected and honored because they were the therapeutic agent for the placebo effect.

Effectiveness of Primitive Medicine Exaggerated

These placebo treatments were not extreme exceptions to rational therapy, but rather until recently were characteristic of most medical treatment. Therapy rested on placebo foundations, despite the tendency of historians to glamorize, sentimentalize, and exaggerate the significance of primitive and prescientific medicine (Shapiro 1960; Shapiro and Shapiro in prep).

Medical historians entranced by the presumed perspicacity of ancient healers are predisposed to cite any substance that remotely could have had a therapeutic effect. In fact, drawing conclusions about the effectiveness of prescientific medicine is an awesome, indeed impossible, undertaking, leading some historians to conclude that almost nothing is known about the effectiveness of ancient drugs (Majno 1975; Estes 1989). The incomplete medical record relies on extant documents of treatment, hampered by difficulties of translation and interpretation, and it encompasses many historic periods and cultures. Since virtually any and every substance was used for treatment and each drug was used to treat scores of symptoms, with each symptom treated by a host of drugs, it is likely that they were all placebos. Because most known vegetable, animal, and mineral substances were used, it is not difficult to identify some treatments with active chemical moieties that could have been effective if used appropriately.

In addition, to corroborate the effectiveness of ancient remedies requires knowledge about which plant to use; what part to use; when it should be harvested; how it should be prepared, stored, and shipped; how much was given, at what intervals and for how long, and with what other substances; for what reasons it was used; and how it was evaluated. Moreover, with the recognition of these difficulties (Tyler, Brady, and Robbers 1976), it is unlikely that ancient concoctions could have been active and useful.

Considering these difficulties, what can we say about ancient remedies that are now often cited as effective: malachite, honey, ma huang, poppy, and acupuncture. The evidence for malachite and honey is limited to weak inhibition of bacterial growth in a petri dish (Majno 1975; Estes 1989). However, if they were clinically effective, it is unlikely that physicians would have combined them with numerous other bacteriologic and noxious substances. Moreover, if helpful, healers would have replaced the more frequently used drugs that were ineffective and harmful, including the extensive use of dung, and if effective would have been used more widely outside of Egypt. Ma huang, from which ephedrine was laboriously synthesized in the 1920s, is the only one of 2,000 drugs in ancient Chinese medicine that can be cited as effective. Although mentioned as a "sedative for cough," it is effective only for the cough from asthma (Chen and Schmidt 1930). In addition, it was combined with numerous other substances to treat many other symptoms and was infrequently used outside of China. Poppy, although the most frequently referred to drug in medical history, is erratically described, inconsistently used, inappropriately prescribed, and usually combined with other substances in complicated compounds that were unlikely to survive months of incubation with dozens of substances, such as in theriac and mattioli (Macht 1915; Shapiro and Shapiro in prep).

Acupuncture, the most extensively used treatment in China for 2,500 years, is still in use, with incursions into Western countries.

However, acupuncture has probably been more harmful than helpful, since it is likely that unsterilized needles were responsible for homologous serum jaundice, which was endemic in China for centuries. Although Veith (1972) concludes that "the maintenance of these cumbersome and probably painful methods of treatment must indicate that they possess healing power," the Yellow Emperor inadvertently proposed a better explanation. "The ancient sages did not treat those who were already ill," only "those who were not ill." His advice provides a primer for placebo effects: treat only patients who are not seriously ill, likely to improve spontaneously, and prone to benefit from nonspecific placebo or no treatment.

Other questionable Chinese remedies include ground dragon (perhaps dinosaur) bones to treat convulsions (although possibly useful for children with infantile tetany); burnt sponge, which contains iodine, for lumps that might have been goiters (Haggard 1933); ground sheep thyroid for goiter and cretinism; and blood-filled liver for blood diseases and night blindness (Major 1954). Breasted commended Egyptian willow leaves, which contains salicin for antisepsis, but so little salicin that it would be as effective as traces of aspirin on wounds. He also thought pessaries of crocodile dung inserted into the vagina was a useful contraceptive because it was ammoniacal (Majno 1975). Although there are no controlled studies, a better explanation is that the suppository was a male deconcupiscent. Other historians cite flyspecks scraped from walls mentioned in the Ebers Papyrus as an insightful use of penicillin; placebos that worked because the stale bread from which they were made contained antifungals; and Galen's pennyroyal for abortions, which became a brief fad in the Midwestern United States in the 1970s, brief because it often caused the death of the mother. Another harmful, often lethal, and unfortunately long-lasting treatment was to dehydrate patients.

Dehydration as Therapy

The overwhelming impression that an extraterrestrial would have of a modern hospital would be of bottles dripping fluid into patients in virtually every room. Yet the exact opposite method was the most frequent, extensive, and long-lasting treatment in the history of medicine (Shapiro and Shapiro in prep). Bloodletting began in Egypt circa

1000 B.C.E., spread to Greece and Rome, increased during the Middle Ages and after the Renaissance, and continued to be used into the early twentieth century for many minor and major symptoms and disorders, and often for routine prophylaxis. Tomes were written about where, how much, and under which stars to bleed. Phlebotomy, with contributions from other dehydration methods such as clysterization, stomachics, vomitives, purgation, sweating, scarification, and leeching, no doubt killed more patients than any other treatment in the history of medicine. The use of leeches was so extensive that in 1827 alone France imported 33 million leeches after domestic supplies had been exhausted.

George Washington, who developed quinsy (tonsillar abscess) at the age of fifty-seven, was probably done in by excessive bleeding, 2.5–2.8 quarts within twelve hours, in addition to further dehydration from both fever and calomel cathartics, tartar emetic, and other ineffective remedies. Thus, another placebo treatment flourished despite its tendency to harm and kill—even dooming the father of our country—without being detected for centuries.

A common underlying theme for these and many other treatments was the removal of the bad, evil, or diseased, both psychological and physiological, which reassured patients, increased their hope, and made them feel better (Shapiro 1960; Shapiro and Morris 1978; Shapiro and Shaprio 1984; Shapiro and Shapiro in prep). In addition, since the language for expressing emotional problems was limited and displaced onto physical complaints, it is likely that psychological problems were expressed in somatic complaints. For example, depressive symptoms could be experienced as exhaustion, abdominal distress, insomnia, or decreased libido, and could be treated with cathartics such as purging, bleeding, and enemas. Religious expiation, on the other hand, would serve the psychological function of catharsis by expressing, expelling, or reducing guilt, conflict, evil thoughts, and unacceptable impulses (as is still done verbally in psychotherapy), and might result in clinical improvement, which could be termed placebo effect.

Although it is likely that ancient healers occasionally stumbled on useful drugs, the inability to evaluate their specific usefulness contributed to their inconsistent use and consequent loss of any benefit for future generations. The only possible resolution of whether prescientific drugs were effective would be to determine carefully the putative name of the drug, its chemistry, methods of preparation, how used, and for what illnesses, and then to translate this information into current pharmacologic knowledge and to conduct in vitro and in vivo clinically controlled studies—a task not likely to be done.

Despite the problem of bias and hazards of interpretation and the claims about the efficacy of ancient remedies, we propose that the available data support the somewhat startling hypothesis that the history of medical treatment until recently is largely the history of the placebo effect.

Nonplacebos in History

Useful drugs appeared erratically and at infrequent intervals. Cinchona bark (quinine) was introduced in 1632 to treat ague (fevers). It was later clarified by Sydenham as specific for intermittent fever (malaria), but its usefulness was compromised by continual problems in growing plants with active substances and by fraudulent counterfeits. Foxglove (digitalis), introduced by Withering in 1776 for the treatment of dropsy (edema), was subsequently established as effective only for congestive heart failure and some arrhythmias. It was inappropriately used for scores of other conditions, such as hysteria and pneumonia, and was plagued by unstandardized dosages until the 1920s. Smallpox immunization and Lind's lemons for scurvy (not accepted by Lind himself) appeared in the eighteenth century (Shapiro and Shapiro in prep). Although treatment continued to improve after the onset of scientific medicine in the middle of the nineteenth century (for example, vitamins, hormones, anesthesia, aseptic surgery, immunization), placebos continued to dominate treatment for the next one hundred years.

Placebo Effects in the Period of Scientific Medicine

Therapeutic nihilism characterized medicine at the beginning of the twentieth century, and although the number of nonplacebo remedies increased, treatment continued to be largely placebo. Even as late as 1950, a probably conservative estimate was that a bottle of medicine was given as a placebo to 40 percent of general practice patients (*British Medical Journal* 1952). Forty-five percent of published studies were uncontrolled and 18 percent inadequately controlled (Dunlap, Henderson, and Inch 1952). Each decade thereafter resulted in an accelerated increase of specific, nonplacebo treatment, with a veritable therapeutic revolution by the end of the century—but, alas, no end to the placebo effect.

Whereas I Was Blind, Now I Can See

The major contribution to weakening the domination of the placebo effect was the double-blind procedure (together with advances in clinical trial methodology). The first use of an inactive substance as a control, as well as an almost inadvertent stumbling onto the method later called the double-blind procedure, was a laboratory study of the effect of alcohol and other drugs on fatigue (Rivers 1908), followed by a similar study in 1912 (Hollingsworth 1912). The first clinical blind study, stimulated by Sollmann and the American Medical Association Council on Pharmacy, was a negative comparison of the effect of expensive natural salicylates with inexpensive synthetic salicylates (Hewlett 1913; Sollmann 1916) followed by a partial double-blind study of opium alkaloids (Macht, Herman, and Levy 1916) and a comparison of ordinary horse serum with diphtheria antitoxin (Bingel 1918). Sollmann referred to the method as the "blind test" for the first time in 1917 (Sollmann 1917) and again in 1930 (Sollmann 1930), as did Bingel in 1918 (Bingel 1918). The next study using the "blind test" did not appear until seventeen years later, when Gold evaluated whether expensive ether in cans was more effective and less toxic than inexpensive ether in drums (Hediger and Gold 1935). Gold followed this with his famous blind study comparing placebo with xanthenes (aminophylline was believed to be effective for angina pectoris since 1895) (Gold, Kwit, and Otto 1937). Gold developed the method virtually alone during the next twenty-five years, using it relentlessly and uncompromisingly in his many studies, and proselytizing about the necessity of controlling the placebo effect of treatment. He called the method the "double-blind test" in his classic paper comparing Khellin with placebo for the treatment of angina pectoris (Greiner et al. 1950).

Although the use of the double-blind method was strongly resisted for many years, gradually it became required for funding of most psychotropic drug studies submitted to the National Institute of Health by the 1960s (later extended to other types of treatment), for approval of new drugs by the Food and Drug Administration at the end of the 1970s, and for publication of scientific papers during the 1980s.

How Blind Is Blind?

The principle underlying the double-blind method is that the treatment being evaluated is identical to the comparison treatment or placebo for all variables except those hypothesized for the treatment being evaluated. To ensure this, randomized drug allocation must be unknown to the investigators, clinicians, patients, relatives, staff, and statisticians until completion of the study and analysis of the data. Frequently, however, the double-blind is unblinded. For example, in our review of 27 studies, with a total of 13,082 patients, drug allocation was guessed correctly by clinicians in 67 percent, by patients in 65 percent, and relatives and other staff in 71 percent of the studies (P<0.01) (Shapiro and Shapiro in prep). The double-blind method can be compromised by differences between active drugs and placebos if both preparations do not have identical etching, embossing, color, taste, or dissolubility (Blumenthal, Burke, and Shapiro 1974). In another of our studies, factors associated with correctly guessing whether patients were receiving active drug or placebo were significantly associated with the type of drug being studied, the side effect patterns of the active drug, higher dosage units for patients receiving placebo in titration studies, patient improvement, and the ability of clinicians to guess correctly (Shapiro and Shapiro in prep).

Present-day Placebo Effects

Estimates of placebo effects are usually derived from studies that include a placebo control group. Because of the variability in studies, it is no surprise that positive placebo reactions range from 21 percent to 58 percent (1,082 patients in 15 studies) (Beecher 1959), and 24 percent to 58 percent (55 studies) (Kissel and Barrucand 1964). Placebo effectiveness ranges from 30 percent to 50 percent in depression (Brown 1992); and when compared with effective drugs, placebo effect is 59 percent as effective as tricyclic antidepressants (93 studies), 62 percent as effective as lithium (13 studies), 58 percent as effective as nonpharmacologic treatment of insomnia, and 54 percent to 56 percent as effective as injected morphine and common analgesics (22 studies) (Evans 1985).

Surgery is especially prone to placebo effects, since controlled studies are not required by government agencies. Some examples are hysterectomy for wandering uteri or hysteria and neuroses, colectomy to remove Bacillus epilepticus from constipated bowels thought to cause epilepsy (26 papers from 1910 to 1927), tonsillectomy, sympathectomy, and gastric freezing. Ligation of the mammary artery to stimulate collateral circulation for the treatment of anginal pain was in vogue from 1955 to 1960 after two uncontrolled studies reported 68 percent and 91 percent improvement (N=120), but it rapidly disappeared after two controlled studies reported improvement in 67 percent of 21 patients whose mammary arteries had been ligated and in 71 percent of 14 patients treated with a sham skin incision. In a recent survey of surgery for lumbar disc disease, although no disc herniation was present in 346 patients (negative surgical exploration), complete relief of sciatica occurred in 37 percent and from back pain in 43 percent. In another study of back pain, 20 percent to 40 percent of patients had decreased pain and improved functioning when treated with sham transcutaneous electrical stimulation and hot packs (Turner et al. 1994).

Placebo effect percentages are lowest in double-blind studies, higher in single-blind studies, and highest in uncontrolled clinical reports of a treatment believed to be effective but subsequently shown to be ineffective or a placebo. The highest percentages occur in uncontrolled clinical reports because placebo mechanisms are maximized. Reviews of enthusiastically endorsed but later abandoned treatments reported an average improvement in 82 percent of patients treated for angina pectoris and in 70 percent for a series of recent medical treatments (Bensen and McCallike 1979; Roberts et al. 1993). Higher percentages of improvement are particularly common for the treatment of diseases that do not exist and in illnesses whose symptoms wax, wane, fluctuate, and spontaneously remit, as do most symptoms and illnesses. Although the percentages decrease for serious illness with infrequent spontaneous remissions, they still appear in anecdotal reports and placebo controls in studies, even for malignancies.

Placebo Effects In Psychotherapy

With increased emphasis on rationality, understanding, and open discussion of intellectual issues and psychological distress, psychoanalysis and psychotherapy became the institutional outlet for psychological problems and placebo effects (Shapiro and Morris 1978; Shapiro and Shapiro 1984; Shapiro and Shapiro in prep). For psychoanalysis, the reliability and validity of psychoanalytic interpretations have not been demonstrated, and a controlled study of their efficacy has never been done. Although many studies report psychotherapy as more effective than placebo, placebo controls are usually inadequate. For example, a monthly 20-minute supportive discussion is an inadequate placebo control for weekly 50-minute psychotherapy sessions, since it fails to ensure identical treatment conditions for both groups. In fact, an inadequate placebo control may guarantee that psychotherapy is reported as more effective than the control. A method of bypassing the difficulty of selecting an adequate placebo control for studies of psychotherapy is to pit one therapy against another, such as Freudian compared with Jungian psychoanalysis, psychoanalytic therapy compared with behavior therapy, cognitive therapy with expressing feelings therapy, and psychotherapy by expert psychotherapists compared with personable college faculty. Seven such studies have been done, all failing to support the superiority of one therapy over the other. Moreover, most studies report that the training and experience of therapists, types of problems, brief or longer sessions, number of sessions, and duration of therapy do not result in different therapeutic effects. The repeated repackaging of types of psychotherapy, now exceeding 250 schools (Parloff 1982), indicates an absence of data supporting the theories and efficacy of any particular school. As Garrison (1921) wisely observed, usually when many different therapies are used to treat the same illness or when one therapy is used to treat many different illnesses, we still know very little about how to treat effectively. Finally, nonspecific therapeutic factors outweigh potential, but not yet identified, specific features postulated by different psychotherapeutic theories, orientations, and schools. Psychotherapy appears to be an unsystematic myriad of nonspecific elements mixed together in the hope that some will be effective. This, at least, was the conclusion of Janet (1925) who noted in 1925 that "it is a sort of psychological theriac . . . one should not be surprised if they do not always succeed, or that such treatments are considered as lotteries by official science."

Although there is general agreement that psychotherapy is useful, beneficial, and effective for many patients, as is true of many notable placebo treatments, the knotty question remains—is psychotherapy more than placebo?

Fraud, Faith, Fallacies, and Fads

When a treatment is a placebo, it is very easy to counterfeit. Fraud, faith, fallacies, and fads then flourish. Anyone can use the treatment because successful outcome is based on the placebo effect.

The power of the placebo effect is reflected in the ubiquity of fraud (quackery, $30 billion annually), faith (religious and psychic healing), fallacies (vitamins, organic diets, excessive jogging, holistic treatment, and alternative treatment, $13.9 billion annually), and fads (new age, lifestyle change or self-help modalities, such as ecotherapy or communing with nature and meditative immunotherapy, to encourage the growth and strength of good white blood cells and destroy malignant cells) (Rosen 1971; Young 1992; Eisenberg et al. 1993). Despite the reasonable expectation that the use of these therapies would decrease as scientific knowledge increased, these therapies continue to appear, disappear, and reappear in slightly different guises, as in a witch's bubbling caldron. The unending replacement of one quackery with another has led to despair about its ever ending (Young 1992); and the continued prevalence of faith and psychic healing (with 15,000 healers in England and 20,000 in France) has led to the despondent conclusion that "The only man with a right to the last word on faith healing . . . would be the last man on earth." (Rosen 1971, p. 176).

Placebo Effect of the Placebo

Successful therapies inevitably become associated with placebo effects. And there is no reason why placebo effects should not also become associated with the placebo itself. Formerly a pejorative word and unethical treatment, with its use commonly attributed to other physicians (Shapiro and Struening 1973a), the placebo has recently become a respectable term and treatment. With growing appreciation of the healing power of the placebo, its therapeutic power, as is true of all therapies, has become exaggerated. Faith in the power of the placebo has become a bandwagon effect (Kety 1961). When this situation occurs, the therapeutic power of the placebo and the placebo effect increase.

The author of a recent best-seller, for example, describes a placebo treatment (laughing at Marx brothers' movies) as a cure for an ill-defined illness from which he recovered; his recovery set him on a path of crusading about a holistic health philosophy as a natural apothecary for the treatment of illness. Without either medical or scientific qualifications, he was regardless appointed senior lecturer and adjunct professor in the School of Medicine, Department of Psychiatry and Behavioral Sciences at the University of California at Los Angeles (Cousins 1979).

Current beliefs about megavitamins, good nutrition, and organic foods (Armaroli 1982; Stave 1982), stress reduction, jogging, holistic medicine, and even the concept of behavioral health may be examples of recent popular placebos, since the evidence demonstrating that these techniques are clinically useful or effective is inadequate. Many psychotherapists believe that the placebo effect does not apply to psychotherapy, since both placebo and psychotherapy are psychological procedures, and psychotherapy is characterized as the ultimate placebo.

Belief in the positive effect of placebos extends even to biological psychiatry. Patients applying to a prominent university study center for the treatment of depression are informed that if they get better on placebo, it means that the placebo had a beneficial effect on their neurotransmitters, certainly a preposterously premature conclusion that exploits the credulity of patients volunteering for treatment in such a study.

This explanation to patients may be based on provocatively interesting studies (Levine, Gordon, and Fields 1978; Levine et al. 1981; Levine and Gordon 1984; Fields 1994) and on other studies supporting the hypothesis that placebos decrease pain by increasing endogenous opioids. However, these studies, which are difficult to interpret and often are inadequately replicated, may explain some but not all types of analgesia. Further, the studies have not been evaluated for the effect of other intervening psychological variables such as fear and anxiety; the mechanism has not been clearly identified; and no evidence has been provided supporting a relationship of the opioid system to placebo effects other than for analgesia (Grevert and Goldstein 1985; Fields 1994).

Another reflection of the placebo's popularity is the current interest in mind-body relationships. It includes speculation about the association of stress, depression, social isolation, personality, and psychological and psychosocial factors on the body. An extension of these speculations is that placebos, nonspecific behavioral therapies, and improved immunological functioning can reduce the risk, onset, course, morbidity, and mortality of infections, heart attacks, autoimmune disorders, and cancer.[1]

A burgeoning literature exploring these issues demonstrates that nonspecific therapeutic procedures improve compliance with medical management, mood, coping, and other psychosocial factors, which are reported to prolong survival from cancer in some but not in other studies.[2] These nonspecific treatments, like placebos, reduce the reaction to distress, decrease depression, demoralization, and hopelessness, and may promote health-enhancing behavior, thus secondarily having a favorable effect on illness (Beecher 1959; Shapiro and Shapiro 1984; Frank and Frank 1991). Increase in survival, therefore, may be related primarily to psychosocial intervening variables such as compliance with medical mangement; improved diet, exercise, and sleep; abstinence from alcohol, smoking, addictive, nonaddictive, and neuroleptic drugs; increased assertiveness with doctors about treatment and the ability to cope more adequately with illness.[3]

In addition, whether placebos and nonspecific treatment have a specific meaningful effect on a physical illness is, as yet, unsubstantiated by well-controlled and replicated studies in humans, free of post hoc analyses of nonhypothesized variables, subgroup analyses, tests of significance done on hosts of variables, and other methodological shortcomings—all contributing to the reporting of chance, nonreplicating relationships (Mulder et al. 1992; Nowak 1994).

Another problem is that the mechanism by which psychological factors, placebos, and psychological therapies affect physical illness and disease is unknown. A proposed mechanism is that psychological factors such as depression or stress can impair immune function, cause or cure illness, and delay or hasten death. Study of these interrelationships is referred to as psychoimmunology. But psychoimmunology appears to us to be charaterized more by creative speculation about the interaction of psychological, immunological, and brain relationships than by critical studies in human beings. The extensive findings reported in the literature are more like neuropsychophysiological perturbations that do not have significant, prolonged, and important clinical effects. Moreover, current data provide no support that changes in immune parameters have any clinical utility or relevance.[4]

Unfounded therapeutic faith based on technical innovations and discoveries illustrates the recurrent tendency for the placebo and placebo effects to be expressed in new ways, much like the previous belief in therapeutic use of magnets. However, adequately controlled and replicated studies, as yet, do not support the hypothesis that placebos have a direct and permanent physiological effect on medical disorders. Thus, we believe that the current exaggerated belief in the effectiveness of the placebo (including myriad psychotherapeutic equivalents) is largely a placebo effect (Shapiro and Shapiro 1984).

Conclusion

The interest in the placebo effect continually waxes and wanes in medical history, decreasing during periods of breakthroughs in medical knowledge and treatment and increasing in periods when expectations are unfulfilled. Current interest in the placebo effect is probably related to a renewed interest in mind-body concepts, behavioral medicine, and alternative treatment.

Medical treatment is less prone overall to placebo effects than are surgical, psychological, and many types of unorthodox treatment. Physicians are more skeptical than heretofore about the efficacy of treatment based on anecdotal reports and uncontrolled studies and generally have more faith in controlled clinical trials. Some of the factors contributing to these attitudes are the requirement by the FDA for carefully controlled clinical trials before approval and marketing of new drugs; subsequent publication of these and other studies with large samples in peer-reviewed journals; the requirement that studies be well-controlled for publication in most professional and academic journals; and the convincing nature of many controlled clinical trials that resolved controversies about the uselessness of vitamin C for colds and of megavitamins for prophylaxis against everything and the usefulness of aspirin for decreasing strokes. Decreased problems with placebo effects in medicine may also be related to the greater ease of doing controlled studies of drugs than of surgery and psychotherapy. Placebo effects may still be a problem, however, because of subtle methodological deficiencies in most studies. Some of these methodological lapses include the breaking of the double-blind code; the use of inert rather than active placebo controls that have the ability to mimic all, or at least most, of the side effects of the drug being evaluated; the extensive use of uncorrected post hoc or group subanalyses; and so on.

Another problem, much more extensive but rarely written about, is the use of placebo treatments by clinicians in clinical practice. This use has come to my (AKS) attention personally and dramatically during several bouts with idiopathic lumbosacral plexus neuropathy, a neurological affliction of unknown etiology that causes axonal degeneration and extraordinarily severe and incapacitating pain that can be controlled only by high dosages of narcotics. Despite this situation, internists, neurologists, orthopedists, cardiologists, physical rehabilitation physicians, physiotherapists, and so on—all competent practitioners—frequently diagnosed the pain as psychological, and routinely recommended placebos (drugs that are ineffective or at dosages that are ineffective), such as aspirin, Tylenol, Advil, many different nonsteroidal anti-inflammatory drugs, Percoset, Percodan, codeine (15 mg), acupuncture, TEMS, ultrasound, warm and moist massage, and so on. Although these practitioners were aware of my research on the placebo effect, when I inquiried about whether there were any controlled double-blind studies supporting the effectiveness of the proffered treatment, the usual responses were such as these: I do not know, what difference does it make, if it helps that's all that matters.

Surgery is more prone to placebo effects because there is no FDA requiring proof of efficacy and of the evaluation of side effects. In addition, controlled trials in surgery are technically more difficult to devise and ethically more difficult to justify than in medicine, such as the use of invasive procedures like sham surgery as a control for transplants. Large-scale examples are the serious questions about the overuse, effectiveness, safety, and benefit of cesareans, hysterectomies, spinal fusions, transplants, and bypasses and other surgery for cardiac problems.

In psychiatry, psychopharmacology is less prone to placebo effects than surgery and overall is similar to medicine. Major problems continue, however, as is evident in the literature, about many methodological liberties marring most published controlled clinical trials. Psychotherapy, whether provided by psychiatrists, psychologists, social workers, nurse therapists, clerics, or other professionals, is the treatment most subject to placebo effects.

Even more placebo prone are the myriad treatments encompassed by alternative medicine, faith healing, and quackery at the end of the placebo continuum.

An unexpected recent development is the new ethical, emotional, and clinical respect afforded placebos. In fact, the belief in the power of placebos has become exaggerated, a bandwagon effect, and the heretofore lowly and unethical placebo has more of a placebo effect than ever before.

Etiology of the Placebo Effect

If everything were known about the etiology of the placebo effect, the terms *placebo* and *placebo effect* would disappear and be replaced by a hugely powerful megapsychotherapy. But we are not even close to selecting the significant from the multitude of variables proposed as underlying the placebo effect, and no more close to using it predictably.

But what do we know about the placebo effect? It is known that there is no systematic approach in published studies of the placebo effect. Almost all studies are anecdotal reports, clinical impressions, theoretical formulations, and post hoc extrapolations of chance significant findings from among many variables in which a placebo was used as a control for study of another treatment. Placebo stimuli, methods of administration, duration of treatment with placebo, measures with inadequate reliability and validity, patient, therapist, situational, and many other factors vary among studies. The consequence is that results vary from study to study and cannot be replicated, making it difficult to compare results and derive general conclusions. Characteristics of placebo reactors reported in the literature resemble a combination lock, each patient with his or her own placebogenic key (Shapiro 1960; Shapiro and Morris 1978; Shapiro, Struening, and Shapiro 1980; Shapiro et al. 1983; Shapiro and Shapiro 1984; White, Tursky, and Schwartz 1985; Frank and Frank 1991; Shapiro and Shapiro in prep).

Clinical placebo effects are not correlated with susceptibility to hypnosis, test of suggestibility, or laboratory studies using volunteers, and vary over time. Placebo stimuli must reflect a credible therapy for the patient. A drug-placebo stimulus would be inappropriate for a patient who likes to talk about erotic fantasies and values psychoanalysis and who would be more likely to respond to a psychological placebo stimulus. Placebo effects are influenced by patient-healer interpersonal relationships and are increased in pleasant, nonthreatening, efficient clinical settings with doctors who are perceived by patients as warm, likable, and interested in them. A positive placebo effect occurs more frequently in patients with manifest or free-floating anxiety and with expectation of improvement by patients, doctors, and staff. Expectations of improvement, however, may be independent or overlap with factors such as optimism, enthusiasm, hope, faith, belief, motivation, and conditioning. A positive placebo effect occurs more frequently in patients who have minor illnesses, symptoms that spontaneously vary and remit over time, and primarily affect the reaction to distress.

Studies of the Placebo Effect

These factors led us to design a series of hypothesis and data-oriented studies of the determinants of placebo effects, using a placebo test combining the reliability of a laboratory test of suggestibility with a procedure that had clinical validity (Shapiro, Struening, and Shapiro 1980; Shapiro et al. 1983; Shapiro and Shapiro in prep). From over 6,000 consecutive patients who applied for outpatient psychiatric treatment, 1,006 who fulfilled entry criteria were administered a one hour drug-placebo test described as "a drug that would help determine how best to help you." Placebo response was positive (decreased symptoms, feeling better) in 51 percent, negative (increased symptoms, feeling worse) in 12 percent, no placebo response (no change) in 37 percent. Placebo-induced side effects (new unpleasant symptoms) averaged 57 percent for the total sample (86 percent for negative, 63 percent for positive, and 40 percent for nonplacebo reactors).

As hypothesized, positive placebo reactors had high anxiety scores; preferred treatment with a drug and psychotherapy or with leaving the choice of therapy to the doctor; guessed the placebo test drug to be the drug that they desired for their treatment; and had positive attitudes toward the doctor (likable, physically attractive, and competent) (Ps = 0.0000). Positive placebo effects increased significantly when the placebo test instructions suggested a favorable response to treatment: "Your evaluation indicated that you should respond favorably to the test drug." Finally, positive placebo response correlated significantly with improvement after treatment with a drug and brief psychotherapy (Ps < 0.0000). None of the remaining 78 variables, including many correlates of placebo reaction suggested in the literature, were significant: demography, diagnosis, past illness and treatment history, previous use of drugs, other symptoms, MMPI variables including social desirability, acquiescence, dependency, dominance, and ego strength. Other nonsignificant variables from post hoc subanalyses were IQ, Rod and Frame Field Independence-Dependence, Eysenck Introversion-Extroversion, Authoritarianism, and Holtzman Inkblot Test variables (Shapiro, Struening, and Shapiro 1980; Shapiro et al. 1983; Shapiro and Shapiro in prep).

Does the ubiquity of the placebo effect throughout history suggest the possibility, popular but hardly testable today, or perhaps ever, that positive placebo effects are an inherited adaptive characteristic, conferring evolutionary advantages by reducing despondency, depression, and hopelessness, and that allowed more people with the placebo trait to survive than those without it?

References

Armaroli, B. 1982. "Rx for Good Health—Nutrition." *Med. on the Midway,* 36:3.

Beecher, H. K. 1959. *Measurement of Subjective Responses.* New York: Oxford University Press.

Benson, Herbert, and David P. McCallie, Jr. 1979. "Angina Pectoris and the Placebo Effect." *New England Journal of Medicine,* 300:1424–1429.

Bingel, A. 1918. "Treatment of Diptheria with Ordinary Horse Serum." *Dtsch. Arch. f. Klin. Med.,* 125:284–332.

Blumenthal, D. S., R. E. Burke, and A. K. Shapiro. 1974. "Validity of Identical Matching Placebos." *Arch. Gen. Psychiatry,* 31:214–215.

British Medical Journal. 1952. Editorial—"The Bottle of Medicine." 1:149.

Brown, W. A., M. F. Johnson, and M. G. Chen. 1992. "Clinical Features of Depressed Patients Who Do and Do Not Improve with Placebo." *Psychiatry Research,* 41:203–214.

Chen, K. K., and C. F. Schmidt. 1930. *Ephedrine and Related Substances.* Medicine Monographs ed., vol. XVII. University of Pennsylvania, Philadelphia: Williams and Wilkins.

Cohen, S., D. A. J. Tyrrell, and A. P. Smith. 1991. "Psychological Stress and Susceptibility to the Common Cold." *N. Engl. J. Med.,* 325:606–612.

Cousins, N. 1979. *Anatomy of an Illness.* New York: W. W. Norton.

Darko, F., N. W. Wilson, C. Gillin, and S. Colshan. 1991. "A Critical Appraisal of Mitogen-induced Lymphocyte Proliferation in Depressed Patients." *Am. J. Psychiatry,* 148:337–344.

Dimond, E. G., C. F. Kittle, and J. E. Cockett. 1960. "Comparison of Internal Mammary Artery Ligation and Sham Operation for Angina Pectoris." *Am. J. Cardiol.,* 4:483–486.

Dunlap, D. M., T. L. Henderson, and R. S. Inch. 1952. "A Survey of 17,301 Prescriptions on Form E 10." *Br. Med. J.,* 1:292.

Eisenberg, D. M., R. C. Kessler, C. Foster, F. E. Norlock, D. R. Calkins, and T. L. Delbanco. 1993. "Unconventional Medicine in the United States." *N. Engl. J. Med.,* 328:246–252.

Ell, K., R. Nishimoto, L. Mediansky, J. Mantell, and M. Hamovitch. 1992. "Social Relations, Social Support and Survival Among Patients With Cancer." *J. Psychosom. Res.,* 36:531–541.

Estes, J. W. 1989. *The Medical Skills of Ancient Egypt.* New York: Science History Publications/USA.

Evans, F. J. 1985. "Expectancy, Therapeutic Instructions, and the Placebo Response." In L. White, B. Tursky, and G. E. Schwartz, eds., *Placebo: Theory, Research and Mechanisms.* New York: Guilford Press.

Evans, D. L., J. Lesserman, C. A. Pedersen, et al. 1989. "Immune Correlates of Stress and Depression Psychopharmacology." *Psychopharmacology Bulletin,* 25:319–324.

Fawzy, F. I., N. W. Fawzy, C. S. Hyun, R. Elashoff, D. Guthrie, J. L. Fahey, and D. L. Morton. 1993. "Malignant Melanoma: Effects of an Early Structured Psychiatric Intervention, Coping, and Affective State on Recurrence and Survival 6 Years Later." *Arch. Gen. Psychiatry,* 50:681–689.

Fields, H. L. 1994. "Toward a Neurobiology of Placebo Analgesia." Paper presented at Harvard University Mind, Brain, Behavior Initiative Conference. Placebo: Probing the Self-Healing Brain Meeting, Cambridge, Mass. December 9.

Frank, J., and J. B. Frank. 1991. *Persuasion and Healing,* 3rd ed. Baltimore: Johns Hopkins University Press.

Garrison, F. H. 1921. *An Introduction to the History of Medicine,* 3rd ed. Philadelphia: Saunders.

Gellert, G. A., R. M. Maxwell, and B. S. Siegel. 1993. "Breast Cancer Patients Receiving Adjunctive Psychosocial Support Therapy: A 10–Year Follow-up Study." *J. Clin. Oncol.,* II:66–69.

Gold, H., N. T. Kwit, and H. Otto. 1937. "The Xanthines (Theobromine and Aminophylline) in the Treatment of Cardiac Pain." *JAMA,* 108:2173–2179.

Greiner, T. H., H. Gold, M. Cattell, J. Travell, H. Bakst, S. J. H. Rinzler, M. Z. H. Benjamin, L. J. Warshaw, A. L. Bobb, N. T. Kwit, W. Modell, H. W. Rothendler, C. R. Messeloff, and M. I. Kramer. 1950. "A Method for the Evaluation of Effects of Drugs on Cardiac Pain in Patients with Angina of Effort: A Study of Khellin (Visammin)." *Am. J. Med.,* 9:143–155.

Grevert, P., and A. Goldstein. 1985. "Placebo Analgesia, Naloxone, and the Role of Endogenous Opioids." In L. White, B. Tursky, and G. E. Schwartz, eds., *Placebo: Theory, Research and Mechanisms.* New York: Guilford Press.

Haggard, H. W. 1933. *Mystery, Magic and Medicine.* New York: Doubleday Doran and Co., Inc.

Hediger, E. M., and H. Gold. 1935. "U.S.P. Ether from Large Drums and Ether from Small Cans Labeled 'For Anesthesia.'" *JAMA,* 104:2244–2248.

Hewlett, A. W. 1913. "Clinical Effects of 'Natural' and 'Synthetic' Sodium Salicylate." *JAMA,* 61:319–321.

Hollingsworth, H. L. 1912. "The Influence of Caffeine on Mental and Motor Efficiency." *Arch. Psychol.,* 22:1–166.

House, J. S., K. R. Landis, and D. Umberson. 1988. "Social Relationships and Health." *Science,* 241:540–545.

Janet, P. 1925. *Psychological Healing. A Historical and Clinical Study,* vol.1. London, England: George Allen and Unwin Ltd.

Kety, S. 1961. "The Academic Lecture, the Heuristic Aspect of Psychiatry." *Am. J. Psychiatry,* 118:363–397.

Kissel, P., and D. Barrucand. 1964. *Placebo and Placebo Effect in Medicine.* Paris: Masson.

Lee, M. S., S. B. Love, J. B. Mitchell, E. M. Parker, R. D. Rudens, J. P. Watson, I. S. Fentiman, and J. L. Hayward. 1992. "Mastectomy or Conservation for Early Breast Cancer: Psychological Morbidity." *Eur. J. Cancer,* 28A:1340–1344.

Levine, J. D., and N. C. Gordon. 1984. "Influence of the Method of Drug Administration on Analgesic Response." *Nature*, 312:755–756.

Levine, J. D., N. C. Gordon, and H. L. Fields. 1978. "The Mechanism of Placebo Analgesia." *Lancet*, 2:654–657.

Levine, J. D., N. C. Gordon, R. Smith, and H. L. Gields. 1981. "Analgesic Responses to Morphine and Placebo in Individuals with Postoperative Pain." *Pain*, 10:379–389.

Lyketsos, C. G., D. R. Hoover, M. Guccione, W. Senterfitt, M. A. Dew, J. Wesch, M. J. VanRaden, G. J. Treisman, and H. Morgenstern. 1993. "Depressive Symptoms as Predictors of Medical Outcomes in HIV Infection." *JAMA*, 270:2563–2567.

Macht, D. I. 1915. "The History of Opium and Some of Its Preparations and Alkaloids." *JAMA*, 64:477–481.

Macht, D. I., N. B. Herman, and C. S. Levy. 1916. "A Quantitative Study of the Analgesia Produced by Opium Alkaloids, Individually and in Combination with Each Other, in Normal Man." *J. Pharmacol.*, 8:1–37.

Majno, G. 1975. *The Healing Hand.* Cambridge, Mass.: Harvard University Press.

Major, H. H. A. 1954. *A History of Medicine,* vol. 1. Springfield, Ill.: Chas. Thomas.

Markovitz, J. H., K. A. Matthews, W. B. Kannel, J. L. Cobb, and R. B. D'Agostino. 1993. "Psychological Predictors of Hyptertension in the Framingham Study. Is There Tension in Hypertension?" *JAMA*, 270:2439–2443.

Mulder, C. L., G. van der Pompe, D. Spiegel, M. H. Antoni, and M. J. DeVries. 1992. "Do Psychosocial Factors Influence the Course of Breast Cancer? A Review of Recent Literature, Methodological Problems and Future Directions." *Psychooncology*, 1:155–167.

Nowak, R. 1994. "Problems in Clinical Trials Go Far Beyond Misconduct." *Science*, 264:1538–1541.

Oxford English Dictionary, 2nd ed. 1989. Oxford: Clarendon Press.

Parloff, M. B. 1982. "Psychotherapy Research Evidence and Reimbursement Decisions: Bambi Meets Godzilla." *Am. J. Psychiatry*, 139:718–727.

Perry, S., and B. Fishman. 1993. "Depression and HIV: How Does One Affect the Other?" *JAMA*, 270:2609–2610.

Perry, S., B. Fishman, L. Jacobsberg, and A. Frances. 1992. "Relationship Over 1 Year Between Lymphocyte Subsets and Psychosocial Variables Among Adults with Infection by Human Immunodeficiency Virus." *Arch. Gen. Psychiatry*, 49:396–401.

Perry, S., and J. Rabkin. 1994. Letters to the Editor. In "Reply." *Arch. Gen. Psychiatry*, 51:247–248.

Rivers, W. H. R. 1908. *The Influence of Alcohol and Other Drugs on Fatigue.* London: Arnold.

Roberts, A. H., D. Kewman, L. Mercier, and M. Hovell. 1993. "The Power of Non-specific Effects in Medicine and Surgery: Implication for Biological and Psychosocial Treatments." *Clin. Psychol. Rev.,* 13:375–391.

Rosen, L. 1971. *Faith Healing.* Harmondsworth, Middlesex, England: Penguin Books Ltd.

Shapiro, A. K. 1960. "A Contribution to a History of the Placebo Effect." *Behav. Sc.,* 5:109–135.

———. 1968. "Semantics of the Placebo." *Psychiatr. Q.,* 42:653–695.

Shapiro, A. K., and L. Morris. 1978. "The Placebo Effect in Healing." In S. L. Garfield, and A. E. Bergin, eds. *Handbook of Psychotherapy and Behavior Change.* New York: Aldine Publishing Co.

Shapiro, A. K., and E. Shapiro. 1984. "Patient-provider Relationships and the Placebo Effect." In J. D. Matarazzo, S. M. Weiss, J. A. Herd, N. E. Miller, and S. M. Weiss, ed. *Behavioral Health: A Handbook of Health Enhancement and Disease Prevention.* New York: John Wiley and Sons.

———. *The Powerful Placebo: From Ancient Priest to Modern Physician* (in preparation). Baltimore: The Johns Hopkins University Press.

Shapiro, A. K., and E. L. Struening. 1973a. "Defensiveness in the Definition of Placebo." *Compr.Psychiatry,* 14:107–120.

———. 1973b. "The Use of Placebos: A Study of Ethics and Physicians' Attitudes." *Psychiatry Med.,* 4:17–29.

———. 1974. "A Comparison of the Attitudes of a Sample of Physicians about the Effectiveness of Their Treatment and the Treatment of Other Physicians." *J. Psychiatr. Res.,* 10:217–229.

Shapiro, A. K., E. L. Struening, and E. Shapiro. 1980. "Reliability and Validity of a Placebo Test." *J. Psychiatr. Res.,* 15:253–290.

Shapiro, A. K., E. L. Struening, E. Shapiro, and B. I. Milcarek. 1983. "Diazepam: How Much Better Than Placebo?" *J. Psychiatr. Res.,* 17:51–73.

Sollmann, T. 1916. "The Terapeutic Research Committee." *JAMA,* 7:1439–1442.

———. 1917. "The Crucial Test of Therapeutic Evidence." *JAMA,* 69:198–199.

———. 1930. "The Evaluation of Therapeutic Remedies in the Hospital." *JAMA,* 94:1279–1281.

Spiegel, D. 1993. "Psychosocial Intervention in Cancer." *Journal of the National Cancer Institute,* 85:1198–1205.

Stave, F. J. 1982. "Of Myths and Megavitamins." *Med. on the Midway,* 36:3.

Stein, M. 1992. "Future Directions for Brain, Behavior, and the Immune System." *Bull. N. Y. Acad. Med.,* 68:390–410.

Stein, S., K. Hermanson, and D. Spiegel. 1993. "New Directions in Psychooncology." *Current Opinion in Psychiatry,* 6:838–846.

Temoshok, L., B. W. Heller, and R. W. Sageviel. 1985. "The Relationship of

Psychological Factors of Prognostic Indicators in Cutaneous Malignant Melanoma." *J. Psychosom. Res.*, 28:139–153.

Turner, J. A., R. A. Deyo, J. D. Loeser, M. Von Korff, and W. E. Fordyce. 1994. "The Importance of Placebo Effects in Pain Treatment and Research." *JAMA*, 271:1609–1614.

Tyler, V. E., L. R. Brady, and J. E. Robbers. 1976. *Pharmacology*, 7th. ed. Philadelphia: Lea and Febiger.

Veith, I. 1972. *The Yellow Emperor's Classic of Internal Medicine,* new ed. Berkeley, Calif.: University of California Press.

Watson, G. 1966. *New Series: Theriac and Mithridatium—A Study in Therapeutics,* vol. 9. London: Wellcome Historical Medical Library.

Waxler-Morrison, N., T. G. Hislop, and B. Mears. 1992. "Effects of Social Relationships on Survival for Women with Breast Cancer: A Prospective Study." *Soc. Sci. Med.*, 33:177–183.

White, L., B. Tursky, and G. E. Schwartz, eds. 1985. *Placebo: Theory, Research and Mechanisms.* New York: Guilford Press.

Williams, J. B. W., J. G. Rabkin, R. H. Remien, J. M. Gorman, and A. A. Ehrhardt. 1991. "Multidisciplinary Baseline Assessment of Homosexual Men With and Without Human Immunodeficiency Virus Infection." *Arch. Gen. Psychiatry,* 48:124–130.

Williams, R. B., and M. A. Chesney. 1993. "Psychosocial Factors and Prognosis in Established Coronary Artery Disease." *JAMA,* 270:1860–1861.

Young, J. H. 1992. *American Health Quackery.* Princeton: Princeton University Press.

Notes

1. For support of the concept see House, Landis, and Umberson 1988; Cohen, Tyrrell, and Smith 1991; Spiegel 1993; Markovitz et al. 1993; Williams and Chesney 1993. For negative studies see Williams et al. 1991; Perry et al. 1992; Perry and Fishman 1993; Stein, Hermanson and Spiegel 1993; Lyketsos et al. 1993; Perry and Rabkin 1994; and review by Stein et al. 1993.

2. Reported as positive by Eli et al. 1992; Waxler-Morrison et al. 1992; Fawzy et al. 1993; Temoshok et al. 1985; Spiegel 1993. For negative studies see Lee et al. 1992; Mulder et al. 1992; Gellert, Maxwell, and Siegel 1993; see review by Stein, Hermanson, and Spiegel 1993.

3. For example, see House, Landis, and Umberson 1988; Cohen, Tyrrell, and Smith 1991; Williams et al. 1991; Perry et al. 1992; Perry and Fishman 1993; Stein, Hermanson, and Spiegel 1993; Spiegel 1993; Stein, Hermanson, and Spiegel 1993; Williams and Chesney 1993; Lyketsos et al. 1993; Perry and Rabkin 1994.

4. Perry et al. 1992; Perry and Rabkin 1994; Evans et al. 1989; Darko et al. 1991.

Clinical Reflections on the Placebo Phenomenon

2

Howard Spiro

Introduction

A gastroenterologist educated at Harvard in the 1940s, I gave up endoscopy in the 1960s, and so I see many patients with complaints whose source has not yielded to the more intrusive diagnostic endeavors of my colleagues. For that reason, I have had to think about patients and pain, doctors and placebos, and the site of what may be called "existential pain" (Spiro 1986). Having prescribed placebos in what I hope has been an honest way, I will relate some of my meditations on that practice in the expectation that others will provide a more theoretical, philosophical, and scientific framework for our discussions. The placebo phenomenon reminds me of the unity of body, mind, and maybe even spirit.

Pain

To talk about placebos is to talk in large part about pain, for placebos relieve pain better than anything else. Discussion of what they can do depends upon definitions of pain and distinctions between acute and chronic pain. *Pain* has been defined as "an unpleasant sensory and emotional experience associated with actual or potential tissue damage or described in terms of such damage" (IASP 1979). It is unfortunate that the word *pain* is used for acute as well as for chronic pain, because the two kinds of pain represent really quite different problems. Acute pain has well-tracked neural connections, whereas chronic pain is more enigmatic, with its origin elusive (Cohen 1991; Loeser 1991). Acute

37

pain may have modulators, some neural connections going upward to dull pain perception and others trailing downward to inhibit pain at its source. But whereas acute pain has modulators, chronic pain has only translators of what is often the "sorrow that has no vent in tears." Acute pain is a challenge usually accepted by physicians, but chronic pain is a burden and a reproach. Theologians may find meaning in pain and martyrs bathe in it, but chronic pain is something doctors often think that people should be able to shake themselves out of. In her book on *The Body in Pain* Elaine Scarry writes, "To have pain is to be certain; to hear about pain is to be in doubt" (Scarry 1985).

Punishment is the first definition of pain in the *Oxford English Dictionary*. An old practitioner's advice to ask patients with chronic pain, "What have you done that you should be punished in this way?" comes close to the truth, since most of us sometimes blame ourselves for something bad that has happened, letting shame and guilt hide under the blanket of pain.

Pain often seems to be the word that patients use to gain the doctor's attention. By that word they often mean that other kind of suffering, what some call "existential" pain that has no obvious locus. C. S. Lewis, the famed British essayist, distinguished between a particular pain conveyed by specialized nerve fibers and any experience, physical or mental, which the patient dislikes, and which Lewis found synonymous with suffering, anguish, and tribulation (Lewis 1947). It is the latter pain that brings patients to doctors, though we do not often recognize it. Chronic pain is called "wordless" by some commentators, but I take it rather to be a cry in a foreign language. Such pain is a sign, an icon opening a file full of sorrow. To treat chronic pain with analgesic agents is, sometimes, to make mistakes in translation.

The Doctors' Dilemma

Although the placebo as such became part of medicine when science joined medical practice (Shapiro 1960), the relative dearth of commentary on the placebo phenomenon suggests the embarrassment of physicians that we still, only a few generations removed from superstition and magic, have to employ something we cannot explain. Medical practice is split between *science*—what can be measured and reproduced and predicted—and *intuition*—the immediate apprehension of a phenomenon that does not find replication or reason. The placebo effect highlights the dissonance between science and modern medical practice, which has been responsible for much of the criticism of physicians over the past few decades. Doctors look for *cure,* but patients still want *care.*

Fifty years ago, catalogues for physicians still carried long arrays of pills labelled "Placebo." Physicians were happy to have them in different sizes, shapes, and colors—liquids as well as capsules. I was particularly attracted to one called "Eskay's Neurophosphates," a nostrum guaranteed to perk up anyone who just read the label. But doctors in the 1940s were still paternalistic, whereas today to give placebos is deemed unethical. The autonomy movement of the 1960s, built on the foundation of truth-telling, gave the quietus to placebos as it led to a general derision of the old-fashioned beneficent "deception" that placebos seem to represent.

It has been customary to confess that the history of the placebo is the history of medical practice itself until very modern times (Shapiro 1960) but that the ascent of science during the nineteenth and twentieth centuries did away with the need for magic and mystery in medical practice. And yet there is a paradox in the 1990s when the mind-body dichotomy is being erased that something which so obviously works on the mind is ignored. Physicians of former times had more faith in their prescriptions than our skeptical age allows, regarding them as more than nostrums or placebos, at least part of the time. Presumably also, more than a few remedies handed down by tradition had a solid empirical base, pharmaceutical in nature, like foxglove becoming digitalis.

Over the past one hundred years, the model of the physician has moved from *practitioner* at the bedside to *clinician* in the hospital, and in our time to *scientist* in the laboratory, or at least to the *technician* (Jewson 1976) in the examining room. That progression has led to the growing dominance of technology in medical practice, what we may call the *eye,* and a corresponding lessening of reliance on the *ear*—listening—and on the other senses. The practitioner deals with a patient as a person, but the clinician deals with the disease in the patient, whereas the laboratory-based physician looks at cells and their molecular malaise, and the endoscopist scans the belly for pains that hide in the head. Modern patients lose the catharsis that only the "listening healer" can give (Jackson 1992). Talk is, as Engel has reminded us, the only way that patients can acquaint their physicians with the inner experiences that led them to consider themselves ill in the first place (Engel 1992). But biomedicine has rejected this dialogue in favor of images that may bear little relation to the patient's complaints.

The placebo phenomenon deserves explicit attention, however unclear is the reason why hope helps. Although a decade ago, it seemed that neurotransmitters, like endorphins and enkephalins, would explain why doctors can help patients with placebos, the mechanisms remain a mystery. In commenting on the usefulness of placebos, I like to point out that doctors prescribed aspirin long before we understood how it relieved pain; we talked of a raised pain perception threshold, later of prostaglandin synthetase, and then of cyclooxygenase and the arachidonic acid of cell membranes. But everyone quite happily accepted the benefits of aspirin, even when the way that it worked remained unknown. The difference is that aspirin was new and the product of science, whereas placebos are ancient and more magical.

As Peck and Coleman have commented, to locate the placebo effect as a single unknowable "nuisance variable" is to confuse the issue; placebo is a term temporarily adopted to label a group of effects whose specific mechanisms of action we do not yet understand even though placebo's efficacy has been demonstrated in thousands of studies (Peck and Coleman 1991).

Terms and Definitions

Terms always need to be defined. In the computerized *Index Medicus,* the word *placebo* retrieves thousands of papers, because a placebo is used in all randomized controlled clinical trials. But its plural, *placebos,* reduces the catch to under a thousand, to suggest a far more generalized usage. Distinctions between *disease* and *illness* will engage us later.

Placebo as Placebo Substitute in Randomized Clinical Trials

Placebos are given in randomized double-blind controlled trials to separate the effect of being studied or to participate in a trial of a new agent from the effect of the drug itself and, of course, from the natural healing that occurs with time; placebos, then, provide the benchmark for any therapeutic effect. In the 1960s and 1970s patients with an ulcer crater seen at endoscopy were given new agents—the H2 blockers—to find out how well such drugs relieved ulcer pain or speeded the healing of an ulcer crater.

There are lessons in what happened, for there was no tight relationship between ulcer pain and ulcer crater: dyspepsia was quickly relieved despite the much slower disappearance of the ulcer crater that was its ostensible source. Equally important, placebos often seemed to work as well as the active drug; in some studies, at least half the patients lost their dyspepsia on placebos alone. At the end of two weeks, the ulcer crater had healed in more than half the patients given the active drug and in only a third of patients taking placebos; that one observation point provided the desired statistical significance to permit the claim that the active drug, in this case cimetidine, "speeded the healing" of peptic ulcer (Binder, et al. 1978). But at every other period of assessment, cimetidine and the placebo proved equally effective. That finding has been true of many other drugs since. Statisticians often select the best answers to magnify the claims for the agent. Although it is hard to tease out the beneficial effect of the observer in any such study, placebos in randomized clinical trials (RCTs) offer much material for discussion of placebos as therapy, as well as the roles of faith and belief in feeling better.

Compliance

Compliance, the very act of participating in the study, brings a benefit that not entering the study—joining a group—lacks, even when someone gets the placebo. Compliance is, after all, what our parents taught: good boys and girls who do what they are told will be taken care of. Compliance studies enhance the old message of king and clergy: do what you are commanded and you will do well.

How well a patient follows a doctor's regimen has an important influence on how well the patient does (Horwitz and Horwitz 1993). If you are compliant, you do well.

Adherence

Adherence has won out as a term over compliance, doubtless because it ascribes a less hierarchical aspect. Skeptics who consider placebos "biologically inactive" emphasize their surprise that "patients who adhere to treatment, even when that treatment is a placebo, have better health outcomes than poorly adherent patients" (Horwitz and Horwitz 1993).

"Outcome" studies, now all the rage, emphasize the characteristic relationship of adherence to "health outcome" in many other studies, from antipsychotic medications for schizophrenia to antibiotic prophylaxis for fever in cancer patients. In one study of drugs to lower lipid levels after a heart attack, only 15 percent of patients who took most of their prescribed medication died over the next five years, whereas 25 percent of those less adherent died during that same period. Again, it made no difference whether the patients took active drug or placebo (Horwitz and Horwitz 1993).

Whether being conscientious enough to take your medicine is just one more reflection of a "prognostically favorable" psychological profile, whether it is a sign of other good health practices, or whether feeling better is associated with taking medication have all been considered. But increasingly it is hard to deny that giving placebos has a very important therapeutic effect or that being studied, *participating in a group,* is highly beneficial. The implications of this effect for joining groups are obvious. Humans are social animals, even in our grief. "Misery loves company," the phrase goes. Talking gives permission to act, sometimes.

Expectancy
What is rarely mentioned in medical commentary is any notion that faith in what is being done plays a role in the apparent effectiveness of placebos. Hope, after all, helps. How much a patient anticipates improving, so called *expectancy,* may contribute to what is still pejoratively termed the "nonspecific effect" of a placebo. *Motivation* also comes in for attention: those who are encouraged to have a stronger desire to respond may report greater or better effects than those who are not so motivated (Jensen and Karoly 1991). Galen on this matter somewhere commented, "He cures most in whom most are confident . . ."

Criticism of Randomized Controlled Trials
Placebo controls have come in for criticism in the past few years. Placebos are obviously unethical in controlled trials when a proven

remedy exits, depending on what is meant by "proven" and what disease is being treated. The statistical significance of an association so relied upon by the FDA depends upon two characteristics (Rothman and Michels 1994): (1) the strength of that association and (2) its statistical variability. A weak effect with little variability is "significant," whereas a strong effect with considerable variability may not be. Strong effects are of more interest to clinicians, but reducing statistical variability requires large, expensive, and difficult studies; small studies are easier, and placebo controls magnify the differences needed. That is how marginal "me too" drugs get into the marketplace.

In my own field, a host of 5-ASA drugs have been introduced for the treatment of inflammatory bowel disease. The parent drug sulfasalazine is split by intestinal bacteria into sulfapyridine and 5-ASA, currently adjudged (for not entirely persuasive reasons) to be the active component. 5-ASA derivatives have proven more effective than placebos, but the very few studies looking at whether they are more effective than sulfasalazine suggest only their equivalency. As physicians prize novelty, the new agents are widely popular and sell at much higher prices than the old "off-patent" parent. Placebo control trials prove efficacy, which is what the FDA wants, but sometimes they give the clinician little further guidance.

On the other hand, when studies do not have a placebo control, drugs that may not be very much more active than a placebo may be accepted as effective. The placebo healing rate for duodenal ulcer has run from 20 percent in London to 70 percent in Switzerland. Cimetidine proved better than a placebo for duodenal ulcer (with the caveats already mentioned), but when other agents are tested against cimetidine in an entirely ethical way, if they prove as effective as cimetidine, they pass muster. However, since placebo-controlled studies recorded the readiness of most ulcers to heal, studies comparing a new agent with cimetidine may be "healing" ulcers that would have healed on their own.

Sullivan makes the acute observation that placebo controlled RCTs define modern medical practice and set it off from mystery, conferring authority on medicine as a science and separating it from other forms of healing (Sullivan 1993). Placebo controls map therapeutic efficiency as a single path to knowledge and so cast alternative medicines into shadowy byways.

Placebos as Therapy

In clinical medicine, placebos are usually seen as pills, and only much more reluctantly as procedures, in either case originating with a physician. The effect of a placebo, on the other hand, is deemed to reside in the patient as the rather more passive recipient of its power. There is much discussion about whether a placebo is anything given to deceive, even if its physiological action makes it an "impure" placebo whose benefit is enhanced by side effects, or whether its effects are incidental to the intent of the physician, or whether relief comes from the color or shape of the pill or from something else equally symbolic. Obviously, receiving any pill from a concerned physician in a medical setting will bring some beneficial effect, especially to the patient who has taken some pains to come a distance for consultation or help. Ceremony has its therapeutic role, as so many successful physicians have recognized.

Things quickly grow very complex. To define placebos as "intentional" or "unintentional" makes their definition depend upon the knowledge of the physician, a somewhat paradoxical and slippery approach. For clinicians, Shapiro's definition will do: "A placebo is a pill deemed inactive by a physician but given to relieve the complaint of the patient" (Shapiro 1960). Placebos may also be procedures, diagnostic or therapeutic endeavors that the physician "knows" bring no pharmacological benefit. By most definitions a placebo must be given by a physician who believes that the drug prescribed is "inactive" by pharmacologic standards. This leaves us in the awkward position of claiming that a drug which is a placebo for one physician may not be for another.

How placebos are defined will depend on the cultural setting and the times, the knowledge of the doctor, and the way that disease is defined. One person's placebo is another's active agent. The definition will also depend on how doctors choose the metaphors for what they do and what they are, the balance between parentalism and autonomy, and much more.

A purely pharmacological definition of placebos that ignores the social-cultural milieu and the physician-patient relationship seems a self-defeating approach, since a medical visit involves both a doctor and a patient.

Disease and Illness

Ultimately, patients feel better, or at least one hopes so, but then we have to locate and define the placebo-effect. To do so, we must distinguish between *disease* and *illness* in the blurred borders between mind and brain. For most physicians, *disease* is what the doctor sees and finds, *illness* is what the patient feels and suffers. Disease is the stomach ulcer, illness the dyspepsia that it may bring. Suffering has a part in illness, along with anxiety. As emphasized earlier, acute pain represents tissue damage, but much chronic pain seems to me to represent a symbol, translated more from anguish than from anything else. Philip Aries saw styles in suffering: hysteria, which was prevalent in Charcot's time, disappeared when Freud made neurosis more popular (Micale 1993). That situation, of course, had to do with what the doctors decided to call diseases. Popular practitioners, particularly "on the fringe," more than rarely satisfy patients by giving a name to their complaints, by turning illness into disease. Undifferentiated abdominal pain, with no apparent or elicitable relation to pathophysiology, often seems to me to be the 1990s equivalent of nineteenth-century hysteria, hidden in the belly rather than worn on (or by) the arm or other parts of the motor apparatus.

It is not easy to separate *disease* from *illness,* given the fuzzy borders between "organic" and "functional" problems. The irritable bowel provides a good example from my field: many people have deranged bowel function that common sense tells them is a normal, or at least a usual, reaction to the stresses of life and the food that they eat. For them, as for many physicians, the irritable bowel is recognized by symptoms in a surrounding sociocultural matrix. Many deem it a response to life, not a disease. But if such patients worry that they have a disease, they will find physicians eager to study them intensively; such doctors will decorate the complaints with special wave patterns that can be duly unrolled on strips of paper and passed from hand to hand to justify the complaints as a disease. Many doctors look for specific "markers" for disease and, if one can be found, do not ask whether it is cause or effect.

Of course, someone has suggested, "Illness, like a work of art, can be understood from multiple perspectives." We physicians prefer molecular explanations to the cultural ones of anthropologists. The different types of knowledge bear on the differences between disease and illness, but for now I will remain with the medical definitions.

Let me assert that placebos help illness, they relieve pain, but they do not cure disease. I have examined the claims for placebos helping cancer and other diseases, but I have found not one placebo that stands up to scrutiny. To make that assertion, of course, I have to be careful about the definition of disease: where do you put high blood pressure, which represents a spectrum of response rather than a specific entity? Hypertension can be helped by many approaches.

The Placebo Drama

Let us look at the placebo drama: the physician gives what he or she believes to be an inert material to a sick person with a complaint that may, or may not, originate in a biologically detectable disease; and afterwards there is the "placebo effect," and the patient feels better.

The placebo drama has three actors, the three Ps: the physician, the placebo, and the patient. Taking them up in order, we must recognize that the patient is the star, not merely the stage.

The Physician

Physicians have faith that every pain will have a site in the body, the so-called "anatomo-clinical gaze." "Where do you hurt?" the gastroenterologist asked the neurologist with belly pain, and was astonished when the patient replied, "In my head, of course!"

For the relief of pain, physicians usually try the weakest agents first, and that method is how they used to think of placebos even if current physicians have so little faith in themselves that they are unlikely to use placebos at all. The physician may give a placebo as (1) a *gift* to relieve pain or to treat a complaint that seems to have no objective explanation; (2) a *challenge* to prove that the patient is wrong ("See, if a sugar pill has helped you, it is all in your mind!"); and, finally, (3) *ransom* to get rid of a demanding patient too difficult to deal with. Placebos benefit patients, regardless of the mood in which the doctor prescribes them—and that benefit is one of their wonders.

Placebos, in a sense, benefit physicians too by giving them what they take to be a harmless way to please the patient. A deeper benefit, making us doctors aware of the importance of mind and spirit to body, is only rarely considered.

Today, of course, most medicines are given with apparent scientific rationale, as physicians have come to rely much less on themselves as therapeutic agents than on the pills and procedures available to them. The very notion of physician as "healer" embarrasses most doctors. "Heal," so common a word in self-help movements, implies something going on from within, whereas "cure" has to do with what the doctor can do to help the patients; we doctors prefer "cure" to "heal." The old phrase captures the difference: "We dress the wound, God heals it."

Physicians used to think of themselves as parents, scientists, soldiers, or something else, but in an era of managed care they have come to see themselves largely as conduits of power only, and increasingly as one unit interchangeable with any other. RCTs have done the same in holding all physicians as equal in trials, to suggest implicitly that the specific physician does not matter. The placebo effect and the benefit it brings should make us all once again regard physicians as potentially active healing agents, however idiosyncratic and differing their personalities.

Taking the placebo seriously, "in the same way as we would any other treatment," some British observers suggest how physicians can reinforce the conditioned response that they consider the primary effects of placebos; they recommend kindness and beneficence and even what might be taken as "marketing maneuvers" ("improve publicity about successes, and suppress publicity about complaints"). But even though they praise self-healing and putting the patient in control, their approach is completely parentalistic. The act of listening, for example, plays no large role in their projected program, even if "silence is a gift of valuable time" (Chaput de Saintonge and Herxheimer 1994).

The Placebo

Deciding on the difference between an "impure" and a "pure" placebo depends on the doctor's knowledge of the science available, as already noted. Milk offers a convenient example of the difficulty: the staple of the ulcer diet for many years, milk relieved ulcer pain immediately. In the 1970s when laboratory studies showed that drinking milk raised gastric secretion, almost overnight milk was abandoned as a mainstay regardless of the comfort it had brought. More recent studies have described how milk stimulates endorphin production and epidermal growth factors; thus, who knows, doctors may once again advise their patients to drink milk. Was milk a placebo or an antacid? Both?

Procedures

Injections and diagnostic studies are often placebos in part, regardless of why they are used. Injections are more effective than pills in relieving pain, a fact that must have to do with childhood conditioning: a "shot" to immunize is followed by comfort from a mother or father. Operations are also sometimes placebic, from those early ones for angina pectoris to later ones that remove an unoffending anomaly disclosed by the latest diagnostic procedure.

The Patient—Pharmacology and Faith

The patient who receives the placebo plays the leading role in the placebo drama. Many physicians have forgotten the difference between a *patient* and a *case,* between the person who has the disease and the record of the course of that disease. In taking the medical history, modern physicians usually reduce persons to cases, abstracting away all that is human. The patient is as important as any disease; the patient's symptoms and complaints are—or should be—the ultimate criteria of placebic improvement. What people think about their disease, to what they attribute the trouble, and their value judgements are crucial in determining what makes them feel better.

In examining the effect of placebos, we should concentrate on illness, on what is felt by the patient regardless of whether any disease is detectable. Patients are sometimes loathe to intrude on this comforting division for the physician. A sociologist with Parkinsonism wrote, "I think of the many times I have left my doctor's office taking with me the nonmedical trials and tribulations that are not his concern as a professional specialist. To worry about what I worry about could severely handicap his practice as a neurologist" (Lefton 1984).

Mechanisms and Explanations

Effect or Response

The *placebo response* has been called the behavioral change in the person receiving the pill, and the *placebo effect* that part of the change attributable to the symbolic effect of the medication. Observers need to be scrupulous about defining that "placebo response" or "placebo effect." Some years ago, I found no evidence that placebos helped disease or that they changed the objective, visible, measurable aspects that we doctors regard as important (Spiro 1986). But placebos do help patients with the pain and suffering that the disease brings. They change the story the ear can hear, but not the image the eye can see. The patient may feel better, but measuring an improvement in disease is far more troublesome.

The Bell-Shaped Curve

Spontaneous remission of cancer should not be mistaken for an effect of a placebo. Nor should survival, if we look at the bell-shaped curve: some 5 percent of persons die "too early," while the 5 percent at the other end of the curve live "too long." Swallows arrive at Capistrano unfailingly on a specific day because those who get there early are called "heralds," while those arriving late are deemed "stragglers." By the nature of things some people with the same disease live longer than others. It is only when healers who claim a beneficial influence can predict who will survive that we can begin to consider that placebos— or faith healing or homeopathy—improve disease.

Explanations for the placebo effect operate on several levels (Peck and Coleman 1991): the lowest, that of endorphin stimulation, suggests a purely pharmacological-physiological response operating below consciousness; conditioning theory describes a somewhat higher level, still largely unconscious. Only in expectancy or motivation do we find the matter in the hands of (one should say better, "in the brain of") the patient. In their enthusiasm for molecular explanations, physicians prefer subconscious explanations to ones that derive from conscious decisions of the mind, probably as a relic of the current bias against psychosomatic hypotheses.

Anyone can respond to a placebo; from one-third to two-thirds of people who receive placebos feel better. It seems overly precise to look for characteristics of pills or even for a characteristic personality that might influence the placebo response. Also, anxiety may be an important factor.

Neuroimmunology

Neuroimmunology, yet to receive a firm experimental footing, still may bridge the gap and restore psychosomatic medicine, which is the 1940s term for the phenomenon under discussion. The mind can surely translate its feelings into physiological function: people die of fright or anger, burglars defecate in living rooms, doing mathematics deranges gastric secretion, stress makes the esophagus or intestine squeeze, and so forth. To extend the control of mind/brain to pathophysiologic stimuli is much more difficult, however. It is possible for someone to corner a burglar, but it is hard to control a mob. Consider a stream at the edge of a field: to dam up the stream is easy when the flow is gentle, but little can hold back a stream swollen by melting snow or heavy rain. Normal physiological stimuli may be altered by emotional or mental events, but the raging torrents of disease are as little confined as floods along the Mississippi.

Clinicians, however, have a hard time accepting the idea that mental events may affect physical events, that faith can "heal." That is why placebos embarrass modern doctors, for they call attention to the persistent dualism of medicine and our so recent climb out of the prescientific swamp. The mind may be secreted by the brain like insulin from the pancreas, but "mental illness" has not yet become "neurobiological brain disease," and many hope that the mind is more than the brain.

The placebo phenomenon exists. To show that a pill stimulates endorphins or that a gesture inhibits them, will elate physicians by giving us something to measure but will not change the fact that hope helps. That may be enough when we consider pain, but when it comes to cancer, feeling better is no criterion. There is a difference between treating cancer with placebos and treating the pain that comes from cancer with them.

Time for a New Term

It may well be time, as others have suggested, to find a new descriptor for the placebo. Placebos have been so disparaged, and the dualism inherent in the division of "psychological" or "physical" benefit has been so confusing, that some new term might be considered for the placebo given in clinical practice. One suggestion might be "seal," which suggests the legal implications of a seal to a contract, the sign of a physician's willingness to help, an icon of loyalty.

Then there is the solution—some would call it the art of psychosomatic medicine, of psychiatry, or catharsis—the benefits of listening on the physician's part and of talking on the patient's. Psychiatrists vigorously deny any resemblance of their craft to alternative medicine, yet sometimes the doctors who give placebos live in the same world as psychiatrists, with the same respect for the mind and its power over the body, the same respect for listening. Stress, however defined, does enhance the perception of symptoms. Psychiatrists cavil at any notion that passive listening is helpful, however, for they deem insight to be crucial and psychiatry to be far more than suggestion.

A Tentative Conclusion

The growth of alternative medicine and the resurgence of "spirituality" that has brought popular discussion of angels in healing, emphasize how physicians as care-givers should consider the magic and mystery of life. Science provides the base of modern medical practice and, important for us, the perspective from which placebos should be examined. But there may be some answers that science cannot provide.

As a clinician, I rejoice that the placebo focuses the attention of patients on their physicians but, more important, that the placebo effect makes physicians keep more than an eye on the patient. We physicians must be humble before our ignorance of how one person can relieve the suffering of another. The placebo provides a symbol of our willingness to help, a testimony to our loyalty and to our adherence to the promise of physicians to try to help, to take on an obligation.

Placebos can be the first step in attesting to loyalty: "I will take care of you." That promise may seem overly parentalistic, but it is, after all, what most sick people want.

The Two Cultures

For me, the placebo provides a lens to look at the stresses in medical practice between science and intuition, between what is immediately apprehended and what has to be measured. That split makes physicians unhappy, but there should be no "forbidden questions" for us: medical knowledge depends upon science, but medical practice requires art as well as science. Study of placebos can span the gap between the "two cultures," for its power lies in consolation and suggestion. Some day the billions of uncounted neurons in the human brain may be traced out so that with a modem we can tape our patients' thoughts and patch shattered hopes with enzymatic glue. But for the moment, and maybe for centuries yet, mind and thought and spirit remain more than hard-wired circuits. There remain for now some matters that science cannot conquer.

Patient and Physician

Suggestion should come out of the therapeutic alliance of patient and physician. When physicians listen to their patients as carefully as they now look at them, placebos will prove unnecessary because physicians will have learned again that they can help many patients through themselves. The placebo is powerless without the physician. Modern therapy has made many physicians believe that they are only conduits of power, pills, and procedures, and that loyalty and fidelity are out-moded concepts from an era when physicians could only sit helpless at the bedside. Modern training, which highlights the metaphor of physician as scientist or detective, makes it difficult for many physicians to feel comfortable or useful in the role of caretaker.

The ever-present need of people for some personal connection, for a group to belong to, for comforting words, is responsible for the burgeoning of complementary medical practices that depend upon a connection between patient and doctor. Holistic medical practice rests upon a psychosomatic foundation. The patient's response can be as important as any improvement in disease: the patient with ulcerative colitis, poked and prodded, with orifices penetrated and prescriptions piled up, may still worry about whether persistent bleeding means that disease is getting worse, whether a cancer has been missed, or what horrors the future will bring.

Words

Medicine has become again the silent art that Virgil decried long ago. The persuasive words of Homer's physicians confronted human illness with prayer, magic, and cheering speech, but today's doctors practice in a world of silence broken by the beeps and whirs of the monitors and the beepers. But words from the physician can be placebos. If words can exult the healthy, reassurance and comfort may mobilize "healing" in the sick, even if the process cannot be measured. Aristotle said that a physician who is able with words to have effects on a patient as moving as a tragic poem, can help more than one who sees practice as a technical, silent art. The therapeutic word is, after all, a reality, heard nowadays mainly outside mainstream medical practice. If a story can make us weep, if a movie can thrill us, then surely words from a caretaker can begin to engender "healing"—of illness.

Using Placebos

It is more important for doctors to think about placebos and how they work than to use them, for placebos have really only a very small place in medical practice. Placebos provide a shortcut to the beginning of the healing process—for illness and suffering alone, but only after evaluation, explanation and reassurance, and the launching of a diagnostic plan. Some valetudinarians, accustomed to the behavioral benefit of pills from physicians, will benefit. Many patients need a tangible sign of help, but the physician who prescribes placebos must remember that the placebo is only a symbol of all that we do that we cannot measure. Placebos are used also to wean patients from addiction or habituation and to help patients with pain of uncertain cause. Doctors need not feel guilty when they give out placebos. They need only remember that the romantic plays a part in medicine as much as the rational and that it is very difficult for some patients to take the active role in their own treatment that so many require today. Ritual plays a comforting role for most of us.

Some day the placebo may prove unnecessary even as an icon of the physician's willingness to help, but that event must await the time when physicians realize that on their own they are therapeutic, that by suggestion and persuasion, by words and little deeds, they can influence and comfort. Now, the placebo serves as an important focus for the physician, but it has no power—only a promise.

References

Binder, H. J., A. Cocco, R. J. Crossley, et al. 1978. "Cimetidine in the Treatment of Duodenal Ulcer." *Gastroenterology,* 74:380–388.

Buckman, R., and G. Lewith. 1994. "What Does Homeopathy Do—and How?" *BMJ,* 309:103–106.

Chaput de Saintonge, D. M., and A. Herxheimer. 1994. "Harnessing Placebo Effects in Healthcare." *Lancet,* 344:995–998.

Cohen, M. L. 1991. "Chronic Pain and Clinical Knowledge." *Theoretical Medicine,* 12:189–192.

Engel, G. L. 1992. "How Much Longer Must Medical Science Be Bound by a Seventeenth Century World View?" *Psychother. Psychosom.,* 57:3–16.

Horwitz, R. I., and S. M. Horwitz. 1993. "Adherence to Treatment and Health Outcomes." *Arch. Intern. Med.,* 153:1863–1868.

IASP Subcommittee on Taxonomy Pain Terms. 1979. *Pain,* 6:249–252.

Jackson, S. W. 1992. "The Listening Healer in the History of Psychological Healing." *Am. J. Psychiatry,* 149:1623–1632.

Jensen, M. P., and P. Karoly. 1991. "Motivation and Expectancy Factors in Symptom Perception: A Laboratory Study of the Placebo-effect." *Psychosomatic Medicine,* 53:144–152.

Jewson, N. D. 1976. "The Disappearance of the Sick Man from Medical Cosmology." *Sociology,* 10:225–244.

Lefton, M. 1984. "Chronic Disease and Applied Sociology." *Sociological Inquiry,* 54:466–475.

Lewis, C. S. 1947. *The Problem of Pain.* New York: Macmillan.

Loeser, J. D. 1991. "What Is Chronic Pain?" *Theoretical Med.,* 12:213–225.

Micale, M. S. 1993. "On the 'Disappearance' of Hysteria." *Isis,* 84:496–526.

Peck, C., and G. Coleman. 1991. "Implications of Placebo Therapy for Clinical Research and Practice in Pain Management." *Theoretical Med.,* 12:247–270.

Rothman, K. S., and K. B. Michels. 1994. "The Continuing Unethical Use of Placebo Controls." *New. Eng. J. Med.,* 331:394–398.

Scarry, E. 1985. *The Body in Pain.* New York: Oxford University Press.

Shapiro, A. K. 1960. "A Contribution to the History of the Placebo Effect." Behavioral Sci., 5:109–135.

Spiro, H. M. 1986. *Doctors, Patients and Placebos.* New Haven: Yale University Press.

Sullivan, M. D. 1993. "Placebo Controls and Epistemic Control in Orthodox Medicine." *J. Med. Phil.,* 18:213–231.

The Nocebo Phenomenon:
Scope and Foundations

3

Robert A. Hahn

The nocebo hypothesis proposes that expectations of sickness and the affective states associated with such expectations cause sickness in the expectant. Because expectations are largely learned from the cultural environment, nocebo effects are likely to vary from place to place. Resultant pathology may be subjective as well as objective conditions. Some nocebo effects may be transient. Others are chronic or fatal; an extreme form of the nocebo phenomenon was described in Cannon's classic paper (1942) as "voodoo death."

The nocebo phenomenon, first named by Kennedy (1961) and then elaborated by Kissel and Barrucand (1964), has not been systematically assessed or explained. This chapter (1) formulates a working definition of the nocebo phenomenon, (2) reviews evidence of the range of nocebo phenomena, (3) assesses the state of knowledge of the phenomenon, and (4) proposes elements for a sociocultural theory of nocebos.

A Working Definition of the Nocebo Phenomenon

The nocebo effect is the causation of sickness (or death) by expectations of sickness (or death) and by associated emotional states. There are two forms of the nocebo effect. In the *specific* form, the subject expects a particular negative outcome and that outcome consequently occurs. For example, a surgical patient expects to die on the operating table and does die—not from the surgery itself, but from the expectation and associated affect (Weisman and Hackett 1961; Cannon 1942).

In the *generic* form, subjects have vague negative expectations. For example, they are diffusely pessimistic—and their expectations are realized in terms of symptoms, sickness, or death—none of which were specifically expected (e.g., Anda et al. 1993).

The nocebo phenomenon considered in this review is distinct from placebo side effects (Figure 3.1). Placebo side effects occur when expectations of healing produce sickness, however minor; a positive expectation has a negative outcome. For example, a rash that occurs following administration of a placebo remedy may be a placebo side effect. Placebo side effects are numerous and common (Rosenzweig, Brohier, and Zipfel 1993). In the nocebo phenomenon, however, the subject expects sickness to be the outcome, i.e., the expectation is a negative one. Nocebos may also have side effects, that is, when negative expectations produce positive outcomes or outcomes other than those expected.

When Kennedy (1961) and Kissel and Barrucand (1964) first referred to the nocebo phenomenon, they did not distinguish placebo side effects from the effects of negative expectations. However, reference to voodoo death, for example, as an instance of the placebo phenomenon is etymologically inappropriate. Kennedy, Kissel, and Barrucand distinguished placebos from nocebos only in terms of positive and negative *outcomes,* not *also* in terms of expectations. Kennedy's examples are all placebo side effects; and Kissel and Barrucand did not separate examples of placebo side effects from an example of nocebo in the sense proposed here: 80 percent of hospitalized patients given sugar water and told that it was an emetic subsequently vomited. What distinguishes nocebos is that the subject has negative expectations and actually experiences a negative outcome. Schweiger and Parducci (1981) refer to nocebos as "negative placebos."

Several elements underlying the nocebo concept require clarification. An *expectation* is a sense or a specific belief that some event will occur. Expectations may be *conditional,* that is, contingent on the occurrence of certain conditions, for example, "I will have a heart attack *if* I eat foods that increase my cholesterol levels"; or may be *unconditional,* for example, "I will have a heart attack"; *person-specific,* for example, "*I* will have a heart attack"; or *person-generic,* for example, "Heart attacks occur." In the latter case, the belief that some kind of event

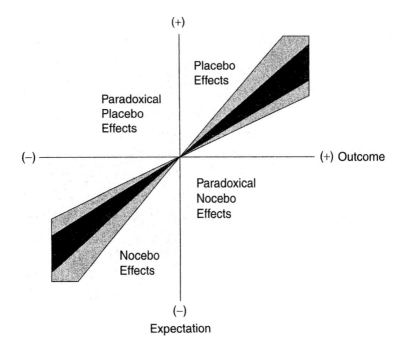

Figure 3.1 The placebo thesis: relations between expectation and outcome

occurs may be associated with an expectation, for example, that it may recur in the future, and *perhaps* to the believer; *pathology-specific,* for example, "I will have a *heart attack*"; or *pathology-generic,* for example, "I will get sick." Hopelessness is a generic expectation of poor outcomes. Expectations may be *deliberately induced,* by bewitching, sorcery, cursing, or nasty words; or *unintended,* by "health messages, eat x/y/z, or else . . . ," statements about possible side effects, or by the very existence of nosologies or etiological theories—professional, folk, or popular; held *strongly,* as a passionate or deep-seated conviction, or dread; or *weakly,* as a casual prediction. Perhaps expectations may be *unconscious* or only *partially conscious.*

Many forms of sickness may be universally regarded negatively; however, outcomes that are viewed as negative in one cultural setting may have a different value in another setting. For example, Buddhists seek to accept the hopelessness of the world as a step in the path of salvation; thus, a Sri Lankan described in such terms should not be thought of as depressed but rather as a good Buddhist (Obeyesekere 1985).

Expectations are not simply logical and cognitive statements but are commonly associated with emotional states that reflect or underlie the bearer's feelings about the expectation. These affective states may play a prominent role in nocebo (and placebo) phenomena. Cannon (1942) proposed physiological mechanisms associated with fear that might account for "voodoo death."

Finally, nocebos are causal in the same way that commonly recognized pathogens are, such as cigarette smoke of lung cancer or the tubercular bacillus of tuberculosis. That is, nocebos increase the likelihood that the sickness they refer to will occur, and this effect is not the result of confounding, that is, the empirical association of the hypothesized nocebo with another cause of the condition. None of these is a necessary or a sufficient cause of the given outcome.

Evidence of Nocebo Phenomena

This review of evidence is divided according to the source or manner of acquisition of expectations. It begins with (1) the inner, mental world of nocebo subjects, moves to (2) their worldview, (3) their nosological categories and self-scrutiny, (4) the process of diagnosis and prognosis, (5) the "labeling" of deviance, (6) sociogenic illness, or mass hysteria, and (7) the deliberate invocation of sickness or symptoms. The review includes selected evidence of what might plausibly be a nocebo effect but for which further conceptual refinement or empirical evidence may be necessary.

Inner, mental world: Mood, affect, and some psychiatric conditions are often associated with negative expectations (American Psychiatric Association 1980). For example, hopelessness is a prominent component of diverse forms of depression. Somatoform disorders such as hypochondriasis and conversion disorder may also be associated with expectations of pathology. Some anxiety disorders, too, may be associated with expectations of pathology. Panic disorder, for example, may involve a sense of "impending doom" and a fear of death (American Psychiatric Association 1980).

Although several studies indicate an association of negative expectations and affect with psychiatric conditions and pathological outcomes (Black et al. 1985a, 1985b; Newman and Bland 1991; Bruce et al.

1994; Weissman et al. 1990; Reich 1985; Friedman and Booth Kewley 1987; Wells et al. 1989), only the study by Anda et al. (1993) uses epidemiologic methods to control for the confounding effects of other risk factors. Anda et al. used a sample of the U.S. population to examine the effects of depression on ischemic heart disease (IHD) incidence and mortality in the U.S. population. They excluded subjects whose initial depressed affect might have been the *consequence* of chronic disease; and they examined persons who were free from heart disease at the outset of the study. Depression was assessed from the General Well-Being Schedule. Anda and colleagues found that persons with depressive affect were 1.6 times more likely to have nonfatal IHD and 1.5 times more likely to have fatal IHD than persons who did not have depressive affect. Considering that an 11.1 percent prevalence of depressed affect was assessed in the study cohort—a sample of the U.S. population—it can be estimated that more than 5 percent of U.S. IHD mortality (that is, approximately 26,000 deaths a year and more than 1 percent of all U.S. deaths) are attributable to depression, independent of other risk factors.

Worldview: Some worldviews and religions maintain expectations and attitudes about suffering, sickness, and death. Buddhism teaches the embrace of suffering/pathology; Taoism advises the acceptance of suffering; Christian Scientists are taught that sickness is the result of delictions in faith (Eddy 1971). Pessimists expect little good, optimists little bad. Few studies examine the effects of such beliefs and expectations on morbid or mortal outcomes. Most studies of the health of religious groups choose these groups, for example, Seventh Day Adventists and Mormons, to examine the health effects of specific habits associated with religious practice, such as vegetarian diet or prohibition of vaccination, rather than of religious belief itself.

Two studies suggest that mortality among Christian Scientists is *greater* than that among age- and sex-matched controls; however, these studies do not adjust for differences in risk factor profiles between the groups compared (Simpson 1989, 1991). Other studies have demonstrated that increased mortality is associated with specific general attitudes, such as cynicism (Almada et al. 1991) and suspiciousness (Barefoot et al. 1987), independent of several other risk factor and health measures. Such attitudes may also be associated with negative expectations.

Nosological categories and self-scrutiny: Awareness or attention to nosological categories may lead to self-scrutiny and to self-diagnosis with the considered sickness. Consideration that the condition exists promotes its "observation" in one's self. A well-recognized form of the effect of nosological self-scrutiny is "medical students' disease" (MSD), casually referred to as "sophomoritis" or "medstudentitis" (Woods, Natterson, and Silverman 1966; Mechanic 1972; Hunter, Lohrenz, and Schwartzman 1964; Ryle 1948). Woods, Natterson, and Silverman (1966, p. 785) define "medical students' disease" as "the development of either symptoms or hypochondriacal anxiety about the disease being studied by the student." They find that 79 percent of students report having had MSD, including psychiatric as well as medical conditions, at some time during their medical education. In most students, Woods and colleagues report, symptoms or anxiety disappeared within two weeks or one month, most often by reassurance from others. In 15 percent of students, MSD lead to "a phobic avoidance of both study and clinical contacts related to the disease in question" (Woods, Natterson, and Silverman 1966, p. 787). Seventy percent of students expressed a desire for psychiatric help, though only 27 percent actually sought help.

In a more common, nocebo-like form of hypochondria—cardiac neurosis or cardiophobia—patients are persistently fearful of heart attacks or other cardiac symptoms, and report chest pain, described by physicians as "nonspecific." A British study (Kisely, Creed, and Cotter 1992) of 108 consecutive patients who were admitted to a hospital emergency room for first-time chest pain found that 66 percent had ischemic heart disease, 17 percent had other organic causes for the pain, and 18 percent had "nonspecific" chest pain. The latter patients thus experienced symptoms in association with their negative expectations. They had a greater, though not statistically significant, prevalence of current and prior psychiatric problems. Patients who have cardiac neurosis can achieve substantial relief of their symptoms when they are taught how to anticipate and think about their condition—suggesting that expectations play a prominent role in the etiology of this syndrome (Klimes et al. 1990).

Diagnosis and prognosis: Brody and Waters (1980) have argued that "Diagnosis Is Treatment." They explain this benefit of diagnosis as a placebo effect, that is, labelling or understanding a condition may promote relief. Brody and Waters do not note an important underside to their analysis—that *failure to diagnose* may have a nocebo effect. In addition, *diagnosis* may also have negative, nocebo effects. Anecdotally, in some settings, the diagnosis "cancer" may be regarded as a death sentence; in this case, expectation may not directly cause death, but may accelerate its occurrence.

Sox, Margulies, and Sox (1981) provide evidence for the placebo benefit of diagnostic testing and the nocebo effect of not testing. Among 176 patients who were thought to have "nonspecific" chest pain not of cardiac origin, researchers randomly assigned study participants to two groups: (1) for diagnostic testing (i.e., electrocardiogram and serum creatine phosphokinase tests) or (2) for no testing at all. Compared with patients who were tested, patients not tested were 2.3 times more likely to report short-term disability (and 54 percent as likely to report that their care was "better than usual"). Negative expectations of cardiac symptoms were thus substantially mitigated by testing.

Medical patients may also have specific convictions regarding their deaths. For example, Weisman and Hackett's study of "Predilection to Death" (1961; see also Cannon 1942) reports that some surgeons believe that operations should not be performed on patients who are convinced that they will die during the procedure. Weisman and Hackett reviewed the courses of patients from one hospital (accumulated during three years of psychiatric consultation in a surgical ward); they carefully distinguished the five patients who were *convinced* of their pending death from those (approximately six hundred) who were *unusually apprehensive* about death. Whereas the latter most often survived the surgery, the former did not.

Labeling of deviance: Labeling theory, a prominent, though controversial, theory of psychopathology, maintains that "social groups create deviance through making rules whose infraction constitutes deviance" (Cockerham 1979); labeling theory has been applied principally to explain the social origins of mental disorders. According to the theory, labeling defines "deviance," including "unnatural" deviance (for example, not looking at the persons you are talking to). The theory assumes deviance is common; everyone breaks the rules from time to time. However, society selects some persons who deviate and labels them mentally disturbed. Labeled persons are rewarded if they conform to the prescribed behaviors of mental disorder and punished if they "deviate."

Thoits (1985) claims that rule-breaking may not only lead *others* to label deviants and propel them into deviant roles but may also compel persons to label themselves when feelings in response to behavior do not fit what they have learned to expect. Thus, the source of the labeling may lie within the socialized person as well as with others. Although opponents of labeling theory claim that deviance leads to labeling, proponents argue essentially that labeling creates deviance. If labeling theory is valid, at least some mental disorders might be nocebo phenomena, insofar as they are created or caused by social processes of naming deviance; mental disorders would be roles that persons enact in response to labeling by self or others.

Evidence for labeling theory is complex and ambiguous (Cockerham 1979; Link and Cullen 1990). Evidence indicates that mental disturbances exist before they are labeled (by lay or professional personnel). Thus, labeling does not appear to be a primary cause of mental illness, though it may be an important determinant of entry into treatment. Evidence from many double-blind studies also indicates that, compared with placebo controls, drugs are efficacious in the treatment of schizophrenia, various forms of depression, and panic disorder; thus, again, biological phenomena are at work distinct from the effects of labels.

Sociogenic illness: Sickness or symptoms commonly occur when one person observes or learns of the sickness or symptoms in others. Knowledge of sickness in others engenders an expectation that one may also be subject to the same condition. Perhaps the best recognized form of contagion by observation are epidemics referred to as "sociogenic," or "psychogenic illness," or "mass hysteria," or, in the workplace, "assembly line hysteria" (Colligan and Stockton 1976).

Sirois (1974) reviewed 78 outbreaks of "epidemic hysteria" reported between 1872 and 1972. Of these, 44 percent occurred in schools, 22 percent in towns, and 10 percent in factories. Twenty-eight percent involved fewer than 10 persons, 32 percent involved 10 to 30 persons, and 19 percent more than 30 persons; 5 percent were of unreported magnitude. (Whereas the largest outbreak noted by Sirois involved approximately 200 persons, an outbreak has recently been described that involved 949 persons [Modan, Tirosh, Weissenberg et al. 1983].) Only females were involved in 74 percent of the outbreaks, only males in 4 percent. Fifty-three percent of the outbreaks involved persons younger than twenty years of age. Convulsions were reported in 24 percent of outbreaks; abnormal movements in 18 percent; and fainting, globus/cough/laryngismus, and loss of sensation in 11.5 percent each. Symptomatology changed over the one hundred years surveyed, from more globus/cough/laryngismus and abnormal movements to more fainting, nausea, abdominal malaise, and headaches. Outbreaks occur more commonly among persons from lower socioeconomic classes and in periods of uncertainty and social stress.

Colligan and Murphy (1979) points out that sociogenic outbreaks are commonly associated with a source believed to be related to the symptoms, such as a strange odor or gas, new solvent, or an insect bite. Sometimes reported symptoms do not fit biomedical knowledge of associations between potential toxins or pathogens and pathophysiology. Persons affected often have repetitive jobs, are under unusual stress, and/or have poor relations with superiors. They may be in poorer general health and have been absent more often than persons who are not affected. Colligan suggests that sociogenic outbreaks in workplace settings are substantially underreported.

Sirois (1975) estimates that sociogenic outbreaks occur in approximately one out of every one thousand schools per year in the province of Québec. A review of recent school outbreaks in diverse countries indicates attack rates of 6 percent to 48 percent (Arcidiacono et al. 1990).

The effects of a person's social environment on sickness or illness behavior need not involve direct personal contact. An association has been found between traumatic death or violence in the community environment and subsequent suicide or suicidelike behavior (Phillips 1974, 1977; Phillips and Carstenen 1986). In this instance, the first victim serves as a model with whom others may "identify." For example, when newspaper or television stories about a suicide are released, the rate of suicide increases in the following week; the greater the circulation of the newspaper, the greater the increase in suicides (Phillips 1974). After Marilyn Monroe's suicide in 1962, 197 suicides occurred in the United States during the following week—12 percent more than the number expected on the basis of "normal" suicide patterns (Phillips 1974). A recent study indicates that teenagers are more susceptible to televised publicity about suicide and that increases in suicides are greater for girls than for boys (Phillips and Carstensen 1986).

Motor-vehicle fatalities follow a similar pattern. Phillips (1977) calculates that, on average, motor vehicle fatalities increase 9 percent above the expected rate in the week following front-page reporting in newspaper stories, and that in newspapers with greater than average circulation, the increase is 19 percent.

Sickness/symptoms invoked: In 1926, Marcel Mauss concluded (my translation), "In a very large number of societies, a dread of death, of purely social origin, without any mixture of individual factors, was capable of such mental and physical ravages in the mind and body of the individual, that it led to death with only brief delay, without apparent or known lesion" (Mauss 1926; reprinted 1973, p. 312). Mauss found supportive evidence in numerous reports from aboriginal Australia, New Zealand, and Polynesia. In 1942, physiologist Walter Cannon, without reference to Mauss, also reviewed such cases, including some from Africa and Haiti; he referred to the phenomenon as "'Voodoo' Death, . . . a fatal power of the imagination working through unmitigated terror" (Cannon 1942, p. 170). Mauss was interested in the power of society over the individual; Cannon focused on a neuro-hormonal mechanism. Cannon had earlier demonstrated mortal fearlike phenomena in cats; Richter later (1957) showed similar effects in rats, though he explained them by a different physiologic mechanism.

Both the logic of voodoo death and the evidence for it have been the subject of extensive debate. Physician/anthropologist Gilbert Lewis has stated that there is little evidence for voodoo death and that evidence would be difficult to produce (Lewis 1977/1987).

Eastwell, a physician, observed possible instances of voodoo death in East Arnhem, Australia, and concluded (1982, p. 17) that "psychological factors are secondary to the basic physical process of dehydration, but both are involved." Reid and Williams (1984), ethnographers who have worked in the same region, dispute most of Eastwell's claims. In contrast to Eastwell's claim that "gross fear," including fear of death from sorcery, is a common psychiatric condition, Reid and Williams report that sorcery is a post hoc diagnosis of death and that dying patients rarely manifest such fear. They also report that patients' families rarely withdraw from care and do not withold water unless it is refused by patients. They suggest that voodoo death is a fabrication of Western observers.

Although doubt exists regarding the validity of "voodoo death" as reported in diverse cultures, there is a similarity between this phenomenon and the "giving up–given up complex"; this complex is also associated with forms of depression (Engel 1968; Lester 1972; Kaplan and Sadock 1989). Patients experience helplessness and hopelessness, doubting their experience to cope or get help; they may feel abandoned and inadequate. "For the hopeless patient there is no future" (Lester 1972). And, as noted earlier, depressive states such as this are risk factors for cardiac mortality.

Although the deliberate study of nocebos may often be unethical because of hypothesized noxious consequences, social psychologists have conducted diverse experiments that demonstrate the effects of negative suggestion on the experience of negative symptoms (Schachter and Singer 1962; Lancman et al. 1994; Jewett, Fein, and Greenberg 1990; Sternbach 1964; Schweiger and Parducci 1981). In one experiment, 47.5 percent of asthmatics who were exposed to nebulized saline solution (normally innocuous) and told that they were inhaling irritants or allergens experienced substantially increased airway resistance (Luparello et al. 1968). The twelve subjects who developed full-blown attacks were relieved by the same saline solution when it was presented therapeutically. Controls who did not have asthma were unaffected by exposure to the same stimulus. (The researchers also refer to an asthmatic patient whose allergy to roses was induced by plastic as well as natural roses.) In a follow-up, double-blind experiment, Luparello et al. (1968) randomized asthmatic patients to four conditions: two groups were given a bronchodilator, the other two a bronchoconstrictor; half of the group given each substance was told that they were being given a bronchodilator, the other half that they were being given a bronchoconstrictor. For each substance administered, misinformation about the substance reduced its physiologic effectiveness by 43 percent (for the bronchodilator) and 49 percent (for the bronchoconstrictor).

The State of Knowledge of the Nocebo Phenomenon

The following discussion provides a review of several obstacles to knowledge of the nocebo phenomenon.

Knowledge of nocebos is hindered by two ethical concerns. First, experimental studies of nocebo effects commonly involve the deception of participants who thus cannot participate with full information. Second, such studies are expected to result in noxious outcomes that, overall, can hardly be regarded as enhancing the well-being of participants (even though the noxious effects may be minimal and short-lived and even though participants may get rewarded for participation).

Beyond ethical concerns, multiple methodological problems hinder investigation of the nocebo hypothesis. Choice of appropriate "controls" to assess the baseline likelihood of the expected outcome in persons not exposed to this expectation is difficult (that is, is the appropriate control a person with no expectation, a positive expectation, or a different negative expectation?).

In addition, several facets of the nocebo phenomenon are difficult to measure, such as expectations, the social environment, and subjective outcomes. Experimenters who inform subjects of what to expect in the experiment most often assume that their instructions are taken at face value—that they are believed. However, subjects may, and likely do, bring their own expectations to such unfamiliar settings. How do the experimental instructions interact with the subject's own expectations? If prior expectations predominate, the experimenters may misclassify the exposure, for example, assuming that subjects have negative expectations when they do not, thus biasing the findings. Persons who do not respond to nocebo (or placebo) effects may not really expect what the experimenter believes that they do. Park and Covi (1965) report finding placebo efficacy even when subjects are informed that their "treatment" is a placebo; but they also report that many of their subjects did not believe that they were being given placebo treatments; six of fourteen subjects had "definite doubts."

The social environment of nocebos is also difficult to assess. Because both exposure to cultural expectations and susceptibility and resistance to their fulfillment may be powerfully affected by social position, it is critical that the social environment be taken into account in the development of an explanation of nocebo phenomena. Using epidemiologic approaches, social scientists have begun to develop appropriate theory and methods to analyze societal effects on health (Dressler 1993).

In many studies of nocebo-like phenomena, it is unclear how much of the observed effect is attributable to expectation and how much is attributable to confounding by other risk factors for the same outcome for which adjustments were not made. With some exceptions (Anda et al. 1993), it is unclear whether the effect is attributable to the gloomy expectations of patients or of other risk factors, such as smoking, drinking, or lack of physical activity that may also be associated with the expectation as well as with the outcome of interest (Schoenborn and Horm 1993).

A critical problem in the control of confounding in nocebo studies is that the "nocebo" diagnosis is one of last resort, requiring a failure to demonstrate a plausible biological, toxic, or traumatic etiology. If a known biological, toxic, or traumatic pathogenic force can be demonstrated, then a possible psychological or sociological cause associated with this exposure is regarded as confounded and not the "real" cause of the outcome.

Diagnoses by exclusion based on current biomedical knowledge are problematic for several reasons. First, current knowledge is always incomplete and imperfect; the definition is thus contingent on current ignorance. Second—and conceptually critical—defining phenomena such as nocebos in terms of the state of the absence of applicable current knowledge implies that as knowledge increases, the phenomenon disappears (Hahn 1985). And third, such a definition suggests that biological or physiological phenomena and (psychological and sociological) nocebo phenomena cannot co-occur; were this the case, there would be no "mechanism" that might link psychological and sociological conditions with the physiological phenomena that constitute health outcomes. The category, "sociogenic illness," is similarly problematic, because it may suggest, conversely, no sociogenic effects in the presence of recognized toxicologic or biologic causes. Psychosocial and biological causation are not exclusive, but rather, complementary alternatives (Hahn 1995). Rather than simply requiring that biological causation be eliminated in the diagnosis of nocebo phenomena, a more appropriate requirement is that biological (and toxicological) causes be eliminated if they are not intermediate links in a causal chain connecting psychological and sociological conditions with morbid or mortal outcomes.

Explaining Nocebos

This concluding section proposes four sociocultural theses regarding basic facets of nocebo events.

First, *local cultures present traditional ideas of what sickness is and of what to expect*—that certain sicknesses exist, with particular manifestations. Because these sicknesses occur, individual persons may be at risk. There may also be expectations regarding the frequency of occurrence of conditions; assuming that I am at risk, the more common a sickness, the more likely I am to get it. Nosological expectations may be further strengthened by etiological theories that explain the circumstances under which and how such sicknesses occur; persons in these etiological circumstances may have more reason to expect the sickness.

Thus, not only are professional, folk, and lay nosologies, symptomatologies, and explanatory models *descriptions* of sickness events—as they are most often viewed—but a nosology is also a *sickness repertoire,* available for performance by those persons who have gained awareness through cultural participation. Knowledge that symptoms such as fainting exist provides a role or script available to be performed. In addition, nosologies may be *licenses* (insofar as they certify the cultural legitimacy of the condition) or *prescriptions* (insofar as they define expected sequences of occurrence). However, nocebo acts need not be—and most appear not to be—deliberate, voluntary, or fully conscious.

In addition to providing a sickness repertoire, cultures have two functions in nocebo processes. Cultures provide rationales for social organization, for institutions, and for roles; they give roles certain values, for instance, highly valuing physicians and less highly valuing janitors. Cultures also ascribe authoritative knowledge to specified roles; persons in these roles predominate in the definition of reality. Persons ascribed authoritative knowledge are more likely to effect nocebo processes than persons who do not have such knowledge. In contrast, persons who have less authority may be more subject to nocebo effects, as is indicated by the distribution of sociogenic illnesses by social class.

Second, *within cultural settings, certain social and/or psychiatric circumstances increase the susceptibility to available nosological conditions*. Role burden, role incongruity, and role conflict, as perceived by people in response to cultural values and personal identity, may increase the risk of nocebo events, which may be experienced as powerlessness. Persons who find their social positions intolerable or otherwise unavoidable are at increased risk for nocebo experiences; this fact could help account for the greater incidence of nocebo phenomena among women and persons from lower socioeconomic classes.

A society consists of a *social structure and process*. The social structure comprises a system of institutions, each with designated roles, including not only occupational roles but also nonoccupational ones, such as parent, member of the choir, or chair of the PTA. Roles are sets of behavioral expectations associated with specific societal positions. Also associated with each role are processes of recruitment, socialization, and retirement, that is, withdrawal from the role. Because different roles are given different values within a society, they are also associated with differential status, power, and access to societal resources. Roles may be critical determinants of a person's identity.

Thoits (1983) has developed a theory of "identity accumulation," according to which roles provide behavioral guidance; therefore, the more roles a person has, the better one's psychological health. "If one knows who one is (in a social sense), then one knows how to behave" (Thoits 1983, p. 175). Persons who lose roles over time suffer increased distress; those who gain roles do not. Thoits acknowledges that this theory should take into account the cultural value attached to societal roles; but she is unable to do this in her own study. Thoits speculates that too many roles may also lead to poor psychological health; however, her own evidence is also inconclusive regarding this hypothesis.

Third, *processes of social interaction and communication power-fully shape attention and perception, suggesting particular experience to be expected.* Interaction may provide a behavioral model for the nocebo response; observation that a particular sickness occurs in others suggests that it may occur in onself. "Identification" with other victims may enhance the likelihood of one's own affliction. Susceptibility to the effects of identification may vary with role status. Interaction, direct or via media, may also more explicitly communicate expected events.

Fourth, popular thought may regard language as a medium for the exchange of information. Beyond this communicative effect, *language is embodied—not only physically through the sound-producing and receiving capacities—but also symbolically, through the power of words to elicit profound emotional responses.* Physiological "mecha-nisms" translate the socio-cultural-psychological into the physiologi-cal. Or, in a less Cartesian language, social-cultural-psychological events have physiological *aspects* (for example, Cannon 1942).

Socially given negative expectations and emotional associations fa-cilitate their own realization. The nocebo phenomenon is a little-recog-nized facet of culture that may be responsible for a substantial variety of pathology throughout the world. However, the extent of the phenome-non is not yet known, and evidence is piecemeal and ambiguous. There is evidence that inner, mental states affect pathological outcomes, inde-pendent of other risk factors; that symptoms may spread in communities by being witnessed; and that symptoms may be caused by experimentally induced expectations. Evidence to validate the ultimate nocebo phe-nomenon, "voodoo death," is unclear. Further investigations should explore the ways in which, like the placebo phenomenon, the expecta-tions of the nocebo phenomenon translate diverse cultural beliefs into physiological processes. An understanding of these processes should illuminate the range and inevitability of these side effects of culture.

References

Almada, S. J., R. B. Shekelle, M. L. Daviglus, and J. Stamler. 1991. "Neuroti-cism and Cynicism and Risk of Death in Middle-aged Men: The Western Electric Story." *Psychosomatic Medicine,* 53:165–175.

American Psychiatric Association. 1980. *Diagnostic and Statistical Manual of Mental Disorders* 3rd ed. Washington, D.C.: American Psychiatric Association.

Anda, R., D. Williamson, D. Jones, C. Macera, E. Eaker, A. Glassman, and J. Marks. 1993. "Depressed Affect, Hopelessness, and the Risk of Ischemic Heart Disease in a Cohort of U.S. Adults." *Epidemiol.*, 4(4):285–294.

Antman, E. M., J. Lau, B. Kupelnick, F. Mosteller, and T. C. Chalmers. 1992. "A Comparison of Results of Meta-analyses of Randomized Control Trials and Recommendations of Clinical Experts." *JAMA*, 268:242–248.

Arcidiacono, S., J. I. Brand, W. Coppenger, and R. A. Calder. 1990. "Mass Sociogenic Illness in a Day-care Center—Florida." *MMWR*, 31(18):301–304.

Barefoot, J. C., I. C. Siegler, J. B. Nowlin, et al. 1987. "Suspiciousness, Health and Mortality: A Follow-up Study of 500 Older Adults." *Psychosomatic Medicine*, 49:450–457.

Black, D. W., G. Warrack, and G. Winokur. 1985a. "Excess Mortality Among Psychiatric Patients." *JAMA*, 253(1):58–61.

———. 1985b. "The Iowa Record-Linkage Study: II. Excess Mortality among Patients with 'Functional' Disorders." *Arch. Gen. Psychiatry*, 42:82–88.

Brody, H., and D. B. Waters. 1980. "Diagnosis Is Treatment." *Journal of Family Practice*, 10(3):445–449.

Bruce, M. L., P. J. Leaf, G. P. M. Rozal, et al. 1994. "Psychiatric Status and 9 Year Mortality Data in the New Haven Epidemiologic Catchment Area Study." *Am. J. Psychiatry*, 151(5):716–721.

Cannon, W. B. 1942. "Voodoo Death." *American Anthropologist*, 44(2):169–181.

Centers for Disease Control and Prevention. 1994. "Summary of Notifiable Diseases, United States, 1993." *MMWR*, 42:i–73.

Cockerham, W. C. 1979. "Labeling Theory and Mental Disorder: A Synthesis of Psychiatric and Social Perspectives." *Studies in Symbolic Interaction*, 2:257–280.

Colligan, M. J., and L. R. Murphy. 1979. "Mass Psychogenic Illness in Organizations: An Overview." *Journal of Occupational Psychology*, 52:77–90.

Colligan, M. J., and W. Stockton. 1976. "The Mystery of Assembly-line Hysteria." *Psychology Today*, 12:93–116.

Conti, S., G. Savron, G. Bartolucci, et al. 1989. "Cardiac Neurosis and Psychopathology." *Psychother. Psychosom.*, 52:88–91.

The Coronary Drug Project Research Group. 1980. "Influence of Adherence to Treatment and Response of Cholesterol on Mortality in the Coronary Drug Project." *N. Eng. J. Med.*, 303(18):1038–1041.

Craig, K. D., and S. M. Weiss. 1972. "Verbal Reports of Pain Without Noxious Stimulation." *Perceptual and Motor Skills*, 34:943–948.

Dressler, W. W. 1993. "Health in the African American Community: Accounting for Health Inequalities." *Medical Anthropology Quarterly,* 7:325–345.

Eastwell, H. D. 1982. "Voodoo Death and the Mechanism for Dispatch of the Dying in East Arnhem, Australia." *American Anthropologist,* 84:5–18.

Eddy, M. B. 1971. "Science and Health with Key to the Scriptures." Boston: Christian Science Publishing Society.

Engel, G. L. 1965. "A Life Setting Conducive to Illness." *Ann. Intern. Med.* 69(2):293–300.

———. 1968. "A Life Setting Conducive to Illness: The Giving-up Complex." *Ann. Intern. Med.,* 69(2):292–300.

———. 1971. "Sudden and Rapid Death During Psychological Stress: Folklore or Folkwisdom?" *Ann. Intern. Med.,* 74:771–782.

Friedman, H. S., and S. Booth-Kewley. 1987. "The Disease-prone Personality: A Meta-analytic View of the Construct." *Am. Psychol.,* 42(6):539–555.

Hahn, R. A. 1985. "A Sociocultural Model of Illness and Healing." In L. White, B. Tursky, and G. E. Schwartz, eds., *Placebo: Clinical Phenomena and New Insights.* New York: Guilford Press, p. 167–195.

Hahn, R. A. 1995. *Sickness and Healing; An Anthropological Perspective.* New Haven, Conn: Yale University Press.

Hunter, R. C. A., J. G. Lohrenz, and A. E. Schwartzman. 1964. "Nosophobia and Hypochondriasis in Medical Students." *J. Nerv. Mental Disease.* 139:147–152.

Jewett, D. L., G. Fein, and M. H. Greenberg. 1990. "A Double-blind Study of Symptom Provocation to Determine Food Sensitivity." *N. Engl. J. Med.,* 323(7):429–433.

Kaplan, H. I., and B. J. Sadock. 1989. *Comprehensive Textbook of Psychiatry.* Baltimore: Williams and Wilkins.

Kennedy, W. P. 1961. "The Nocebo Reaction." *Medical World,* 91:203–205.

Kisely, S. R., F. H. Creed, and L. Cotter. 1992. "The Course of Psychiatric Disorder Associated with Non-specific Chest Pain." *J. Psychosom. Res.,* 36(4):329–335.

Kissel, P., and D. Barrucand. 1964. *Placebos et Effet Placebo En Medecine.* Paris: Masson.

Klimes, I., R. A. Mayou, M. J. Pearce, L. Coles, and J. R. Fagg. 1990. "Psychological Treatment for Atypical Non-cardiac Chest Pain: A Controlled Evaluation." *Psychological Medicine,* 20:605–611.

Lancman, M. E., J. J. Asconape, W. J. Craven, G. Howard, and J. K. Penry. 1994. "Predictive Value of Induction of Psychogenic Seizures by Suggestion." *Annals of Neurology,* 35(3):359–361.

Landrigan, P. J., and B. Miller. 1983. "The Arjenyattah Epidemic: Home Interview Data and Toxicological Aspects." *Lancet,* 24(31):1474–1476.

Lester, D. 1972. "Voodoo Death: Some New Thoughts on an Old Explanation." *American Anthropologist,* 74:386–390.

Lewis, G. 1987. "Fear of Sorcery and the Problem of Death by Suggestion." *J. Sci. Med.*, 24(12):997–1010.

Link, B. G., and F. T. Cullen. 1990. "The Labeling Theory of Mental Disorder: A Review of the Evidence." *Research in Community and Mental Health*, 6:75–105.

Luparello, T. J., N. Leist, C. H. Lourie, and P. Sweet. 1970. "The Interaction of Psychologic Stimuli and Pharmacologic Agents on Airway Reactivity in Asthmatic Subjects." *Psychosomatic Medicine*, 32(5):509–513.

Luparello, T. J., H. A. Lyons, E. R. Bleecker, and E. R. McFadden. 1968. "Influences of Suggestion on Airway Reactivity in Asthmatic Subjects." *Psychosomatic Medicine*, 30:819–825.

Martin, R. L., C. R. Cloninger, S. B. Guze, and P. J. Clayton. 1985a. "Mortality in a Follow-up of 500 Psychiatric Outpatients: I. Total Mortality." *Arch. Gen. Psychiatry*, 42:47–54.

———. 1985b. "Mortality in a Follow-up of 500 Psychiatric Outpatients: II. Cause-specific Mortality." *Arch. Gen. Psychiatry*, 42:58–66.

Mauss, M. 1926/1973. "Definition. De la Suggestion Collective de l'idée de Mort." In: *Mauss M. Sociologie et Anthropologie*. Paris, France: Presses Universitaires de France, p. 313–320.

Mechanic, D. 1972. "Social Psychologic Factors Affecting the Presentation of Bodily Complaints." *N. Engl. J. Med.*, 286(21):1132–1139.

Medical Research Council Working Party on Mild to Moderate Hypertension. 1977. "Randomised Controlled Trial of Treatment for Mild Hypertension: Design and Pilot Trial." *Br. Med. J.*, 1:1437–1440.

Modan, B., M. Tirosh, E. Weissenberg, et al. 1983. "The Arjenyattah Epidemic: A Mass Phenomenon: Spread and Triggering Factors." *Lancet*, 24/31:1472–1474.

Newman, S. C., and R. C. Bland. 1991. "Mortality in a Cohort of Patients with Schizophrenia: A Record Linkage Study." *Can. J. Psychiatry*, 36:239–245.

Obeyesekere, G. 1985. "Depression, Buddhism, and the Work of Culture in Sri Lanka." In A. M. Kleinman and B. Good, eds. *Studies in the Anthropology and Cross-cultural Psychiatry of Affect and Disorder*. Berkeley, Calif.: University of California Press.

Park, L. C., and L. Covi. 1965. "Non-blind Placebo Trial: An Exploration of Neurotic Outpatients' Responses to Placebo When It's Inert Content Is Disclosed." *Arch. Gen. Psychiatry*, 12:336–345.

Philen, R. M., E. M. Kilbourne, T. W. McKinley, and R. G. Parrish. 1989. "Mass Sociogenic Illness by Proxy: Parentally Reported Epidemic in an Elementary School." *Lancet*, 2:1372–1376.

Phillips, D. P. 1974. "The Influence of Suggestion on Suicide: Substantive and Theoretical Implications of the Werther Effect." *American Sociological Review*, 39:340–354.

———. 1977. "Motor Vehicle Fatalities Increase Just after Publicized Suicide Stories." *Science,* 196:1464–1465.

Phillips, D. P., and L. L. Carstensen. 1986. "Clustering of Teenage Suicides after Television News Stories about Suicide." *N. Engl. J. Med.,* 315:685–689.

Reich, P. 1985. "Psychological Predisposition to Life-threatening Arrhythmias." *Ann. Rev. Med.,* 36:397–405.

Reid, J., and N. Williams. 1984. "Voodoo Death in Arnhem Land: Whose Reality?" [Commentary]. *American Anthropologist,* 84:121–133.

Richter, C. 1957. "On the Phenomenon of Sudden Death in Animals and Man." *Psychosomatic Medicine,* 19(3):191–198.

Robins, L. N. 1993. "Does Depression Cause Heart Disease?" [Editorial]. *Epidemiology,* 4(4):281–283.

Rosenzweig, P., S. Brohier, and A. Zipfel. 1993. "The Placebo Effect in Healthy Volunteers: Influence of Experimental Conditions on the Adverse Events Profile During Phase I Studies." *Clinical Pharmacology and Therapeutics,* 54(5):578–583.

Ryle, J. A. 1948. "The Twenty-first Maudsley Lecture: Nosophobia." *J. Mental Science,* 394:1–17.

Schachter, S., and J. E. Singer. 1962. "Cognitive, Social, and Physiological Determinants of Emotional State." *Psychological Review,* 69(5):379–399.

Schoenborn, C. A., and J. Horm. 1993. "Negative Moods as Correlates of Smoking and Heavier Drinking: Implications for Health Promotion." *Advance Data,* 236:1–12.

Schweiger, A., and A. Parducci. 1981. "Nocebo: The Psychologic Induction of Pain." *Pav. J. Biol. Sci.,* 16:140–143.

Simpson, W. F. 1989. "Comparative Longevity in a College Cohort of Christian Scientists." *JAMA,* 262(12):1657–1658.

———. 1991. "Comparative Mortality of Two College Groups, 1945–83. Emporia, Kansas: 1945–1983." *MMWR,* 23:41(33):579–82.

Sirois, F. 1974. "Epidemic Hysteria." *Acta Psychiatrica Scandinavia,* 51(252):7–44.

———. 1975. "Propos de la Fréquence Des Épidémies D'hystérie." *Union Med. Canada,* 104:121–123.

Sox, H. C., I. Margulies, and C. H. Sox. 1981. "Psychologically Mediated Effects of Diagnostic Tests." *Ann. Intern. Med.,* 95:680–685.

Sternbach, R. A. 1964. "The Effects of Instructional Sets on Autonomic Responsivity." *Psychophysiology* 1(1):67–72.

Thoits, P. A. 1983. "Multiple Identities and Psychological Well-being: A Reformulation and Test of the Social Isolation Hypothesis." *Amer. Sociol. Rev.,* 48:174–187.

———. 1985. "Self-labeling Processes in Mental Illness: The Role of Emotional Deviance." *Am. J. Sociology,* 91(2):221–249.

Weisman, A. D., and T. P. Hackett. 1961. "Predilection to Death: Death and Dying as a Psychiatric Problem." *Psychosomatic Medicine,* 23(3):232–256.

Weissman, M. M., J. S. Markowitz, R. Ouellette, S. Greenwald, and J. P. Kahn. 1990. "Panic Disorder and Cardiovascular/cerebrovascular Problems: Results from a Community Survey." *Am. J. Psychiatry,* 147:1504–1508.

Wells, K. B., A. Stewart, R. D. Hays, et al. 1989. "The Functioning and Well-being of Depressed Patients." *JAMA,* 262(7):914–919.

White, L., B. Tursky, and G. E. Schwartz, eds. 1985. *Placebo: Clinical Phenomena and New Insights.* New York: Guilford Press.

Woods, S. M., J. Natterson, and J. Silverman. 1966. "Medical Students' Disease: Hypochondriasis in Medical Education." *Journal Medical Education,* 41:785–790.

The Doctor as Therapeutic Agent: A Placebo Effect Research Agenda

4

Howard Brody

In his 1911 play, *The Doctor's Dilemma,* George Bernard Shaw described one of his characters, Dr. Sir Ralph Bloomfield Bonington ("B. B.") as follows: "Cheering, reassuring, healing by the mere incompatibility of disease or anxiety with his welcome presence. Even broken bones, it is said, have been known to unite at the sound of his voice."

B. B. might be described as a sort of walking placebo. It happens in the play that B. B. is also totally incompetent in the scientific sense; and thus Shaw, deliberately or unconsciously, reinforces the false dichotomy between the "science" and the "art" of medicine. But there is no logical reason why a physician of B. B.'s personality might not be as scientifically informed and skilled as anyone. If that were the case, B. B. would be the ideal physician, bestowing upon each patient the twin healing powers of medical science and his own personality. This improved version of B. B. would seem to have anticipated Houston's title for his oft-quoted 1938 paper, "The Doctor Himself as a Therapeutic Agent"; and Findlay's 1953 comment that "the physician is a vastly more important institution than the drug store."

When I equate the ideal physician with a sort of walking placebo, I am aware that I commit an outrage against the sensibilities of many modern physicians, who view the term "placebo" as highly stigmatized and suggestive of quackery and charlatanism. In their view, it is nonsense to suggest that one can be *both* a scientific physician and a "walking placebo." The negative connotation attached to the term

77

"placebo" today seems to have two primary origins, one worthy of discussion, the other of dismissal. First, the way that physicians have traditionally used placebos in clinical practice requires deception of the patient; and it is the quack or charlatan, not the legitimate physician, whose remedies lose their effectiveness once their true content is revealed. The brief reply to this appropriate ethical concern is to distinguish carefully between the *placebo,* which we ought to use today primarily as a research tool, and the *placebo effect,* which we ought to try to incorporate into clinical practice. There are many nondeceptive ways to stimulate a placebo effect, even if there are serious ethical problems in the use of placebos in routine medical therapeutics (Brody 1982, 1995). Second, modern medicine may cling to a simplistic mind-body dualism (often mistakenly attributed to Descartes) which rejects from its purview any therapy that operates through the mind instead of the body. If this is the reason to disparage placebo effects, then those reasoners themselves must be dismissed as unscientific, since a simplistic, dualist view is simply incapable of accommodating a large body of scientific data which modern medicine has accumulated, the placebo effect being only one instance (Engel 1987).

B. B.'s example prompts us to consider what more we might learn about placebo effects that would allow physicians better to heal their patients. I shall address in the following passage the research agenda that seems to follow most naturally from this goal, considering what we already think that we know about placebo responses.

One final introductory point: it might seem inappropriate to proceed without defining the terms *placebo* and *placebo effect* in a more formal fashion, as I have tried to do elsewhere (Brody 1985). There are, however, good reasons to avoid this exercise and to reply to any serious questions instead by enumerating examples of the actual phenomena that we have in mind. An effective formal definition would say exactly what we mean by "placebo effects" without begging any important empirical questions about how these effects are produced; and this turns out in practice to be extremely hard to do—narrow definitions represent only a portion of placebo phenomena, while broad definitions almost always implicitly import theories of causation and mechanism.[1] Moreover, the working language of medicine is so ridden with mind-body-dualist assumptions that it is hard to describe the phenomena in terms that the average physician would recognize, and at the same time acknowledge the forms of research that I will allude to later. Obviously, confusion arises if one defines a placebo as an "inert" remedy, since if it has no effect, it is not worth studying. Confusion arises in a more complex way if one defines placebo as operating by means *other than* the recognized pharmacologic or physiologic pathways to which biomedical sciences currently attributes drug responses; because as neuroscience research proceeds along the lines that we advocate, who can say that we will not come to explain other drug effects by appeals to the very same neural pathways? It is hard to define "placebo effect" without engaging in a small-scale project to reform modern medical thinking, making the definition useless for the unconverted. This central feature of the concept of "placebo" makes it a problem for writers of definitions but an opportunity for investigators and clinicians.

The Meaning of Meaning

I have previously suggested that a careful review of the empirical data on placebo response, to date, points toward a meaning model of placebo action (Brody 1980, 1985, 1986). A positive placebo response is most likely to occur in a patient when the meaning attached to that illness experience by the patient is altered in a positive direction. "Meaning," in turn, consists of at least three general components— providing an understandable and satisfying explanation of the illness; demonstrating care and concern; and holding out an enhanced promise of mastery or control over the symptoms. These components can be further subdivided for empirical study, if desired; for instance, Novack (1987), in reviewing the "therapeutic aspects of medical encounters," lists twelve separate factors, which could for rough purposes be lumped under the three headings I have proposed.

The suggestion which next follows is that the research program for arriving at a full understanding of the science of the placebo response consists of two major agendas, which must at some point interdigitate but which also require the use of very different research methods. One agendum is to study what counts as a "meaningful" medical or healing encounter for any given individual, at any given time, under specified circumstances. The second agendum is to determine by what intermediate pathways the brain and body translate a perception of "meaningfulness" into end organ changes and ultimately, symptomatic relief. (For simplicity I will not here be discussing negative or nocebo effects; I will assume that once we understand the positive placebo response, through both of these research agenda, we will simultaneously gain knowledge of how the negative effects might be produced.)[2]

Since much has already been said in this volume about the second research agendum, which can be addressed through the neurosciences and related disciplines, I will focus my attention initially on the first research agendum, and next on the less-well-formulated question of whether the second research agendum can inform the first, or vice versa. Can we talk about a neurobiology of meaning? Can a careful study of the wiring diagram of the brain and body give us some clues about how the human mind attaches meaning to various events in the world? Can a careful assessment of which stimuli a person finds meaningful tell the neuroscientist in what anatomic locations to look for intermediary processes?

What Are Meaningful Healing Stimuli?

We have supposed that B. B. is an effective healer because, above and beyond any scientific healing techniques that he might employ, he is perceived by the patient as powerful and persuasive. Further, we have supposed that he exercises that power and persuasion through some specific sorts of actions—he offers the patient either an explanation of what is happening, or perhaps some mumbo-jumbo which sounds like an explanation and which the patient finds reassuring; his manner somehow expresses care and concern for the patient; and he makes the patient either feel more in control of the symptoms, or else to feel that he or she need not worry about control because B. B. has taken charge of things anyway.

What is meant by "meaning"? I follow Bruner (1986) in adopting what is fundamentally a narrative approach; that is, I assume that the most fundamental and pervasive way we have of assigning meaning to things is to tell stories about them. A narrative is a way of situating myself both in relation to some experience and in relation to some other important people in my immediate environment, over a limited period of time. Narratives have two important characteristics for our purposes. First, narratives are constructed by humans and not simply given by the world. Second, they are open to criticism as being more or less plausible accounts of the events and the people in question. (We may add that what count as standards of rationality, that determine which narratives are more or less plausible, are heavily influenced by sociocultural factors.) For my purposes, we can see the question "What counts as a meaningful stimulus for purposes of inducing a placebo response?" as having an appropriate answer in the form of a story that could be told about that stimulus in relation to that person, the person's history, and the sociocultural background.

There are different senses of "meaning." In one sense, we can ask, "What does 'appendix' mean?" and we can then be shown that part of the body which corresponds with that anatomic term, so that meaning suggests a very simple one-to-one correspondence with an object in the world. In another sense, we can ask, "What is the meaning of life?" and obviously no one-to-one association is available as an answer; this sense of "meaning" forces us to look within a concept to understand its function and its logic. I would submit, though the question deserves a good deal more discussion, that the "meaning of an illness experience" is "meaning" in the second sense. It seems plausible that when persons try to construct meaning to explain or understand illness experiences, they commonly relate these to the larger meanings about mortality, the origins of evil, and so on. At any rate, it seems clear that when we ask about the "meaning of an illness experience," there is no object "out there" in the world that could be pointed to by way of an answer. Biomedical science has reified "disease" so that we often imagine it to exist as an object; but it does so only at the cost of removing from "disease" almost all understanding of what the patient experiences phenomenologically.[3]

The meaning model is an attractive theoretical model for the placebo effect. Most of the available empirical data on placebo response is compatible with this model. But, in addition, the meaning model offers the clinician practical guidelines for producing a positive placebo response in the patient. Of all the various actions B. B. might engage in, the meaning model signals which ones are most likely to be responsible for a healing effect. And, if some of B. B.'s behavior is either scientifically or ethically unsound (such as, for example, involving patient deception), the meaning model helps us to discover appropriate substitutes which will elicit a healing effect through more appropriate means.

But the power and persuasion of B. B.'s actions imply, at least in part, a set of social and cultural preconditions. Perhaps if we could magically transport B. B. into a totally foreign culture, which had never heard the English language and knew nothing of English medicine or social practices, B. B. might still be seen by onlookers as a powerful and persuasive personage, perhaps because he has a deep, booming voice and a large stature, for instance. However, we would find it hard to imagine B. B.'s assuming the role of a *healer* in that foreign culture with any degree of facility—unless he somehow managed to produce healing effects purely through the sense of radical difference between his world and the world of that culture. (Compare, for example, the popularity of "Indian" cures in American nineteenth-century patent medicine advertisements, or the popularity of acupuncture in the U. S. today.)

B. B. is able to impress English patients because they have been preconditioned by social and cultural experiences to attribute a certain meaning or significance to particular practices and behaviors. To mention just one example: B. B. can apply two aspects of healing simultaneously when he provides a soothing explanation for an illness, because the usual patient is likely to assume that the ability to explain something carries with it a power to control that phenomenon. But that assumption is hardly independent of culture. Rather, it is typical of the Western post-Enlightenment culture at a certain time in history to believe that science can exercise power over the natural world and that it does so in part by naming and categorizing natural phenomena. I will leave to my anthropologist colleagues the question of how closely or distantly related this Western cultural trait might be to magical belief systems in other cultures, in which words, spoken under the right circumstances by the right person, may be seen as having magical powers to alter natural events.

Here is another example: B. B.'s patients see him as a powerful figure, and this vision enhances the likelihood that they will find his explanations acceptable and informative and will feel that the illness is likely to submit itself to his control. But that perception of power is highly contingent upon B. B.'s status in society, which is linked to his title and family ties, his wealth, the sort of education he received, the clothes he wears, and in what type of vehicle he rides on his daily rounds. Moreover, besides the social power implicit in family, education, and wealth, B. B. wields an important cultural power, to the extent that English society has come to view the medical profession as having a privileged access to "the truth" about certain aspects of human function. In this regard, we might say of B. B. what Kleinman and Sung (1976) have said in rather stronger terms about folk healers in Taiwan: on the basis of how that culture defines the healers' role in healing practices, the patient who submits to their care and experiences the proper rituals *must* be healed; to go on believing that one is sick afterward is tantamount to declaring that one is no longer a part of the Taiwanese culture. (Typically, in such situations, an apparent therapeutic failure may be explained through some sort of noncompliance or failure to believe or participate fully in the healing ceremony; or a sufferer may report himself or herself as having been cured of the disease even though, upon questioning, the person will admit to a continuation of many of the same symptoms.) In sum, it seems that the scientific study of society and culture will play an essential role in explaining to us what sorts of actions and behaviors are seen as "meaningful" by various people in various circumstances.

While a psychology focused upon the individual as a discrete unit may miss important aspects of the social and cultural environment which are necessary to explain "meaning," we are nevertheless left with important psychological questions. Some that currently seem important to me are the relative importance, for the placebo response, of human cognition, emotion, and unconscious processes. These questions, in turn, begin to anticipate the next important concern, which is how the two large research agenda—the "mechanistic" and the "meaning"-oriented agenda—might inform each other in the end.

Some important recent research has focused upon conditioning theory as a predictor of placebo responses. At first glance, it would appear that these research findings are seriously at odds with the meaning model. The model seems to require that human cognition is an important intermediary process, first, in determining that various external stimuli are "meaningful" and, hence, in triggering whatever neurological, immunological, or biochemical pathway or pathways turn out to be implicated in placebo effects. But if the rat model is an appropriate experimental tool for elucidating conditioned responses to various medications, then either rats think about their world in a more sophisticated way than we have previously realized or else cognition is much less important in producing the placebo response than the meaning model would hold to be the case.

However, the papers by Ader and Kirsch in this volume make clear that conditioning theory has moved beyond classical conditioning so as to include a place for cognitive processing of information. Indeed, the suggestion that all treatment protocols in human medicine may be viewed as a reinforcement schedule from a conditioning standpoint offers some valuable research suggestions for primary care medicine. For instance, one aspect of primary care that has been little explored in an empirically rigorous fashion is at what point the physician should ask the patient to return for a subsequent visit during any one of a number of common illness or chronic disease processes. It seems worth studying this question, viewing the scheduling of return visits—even those that do not involve explicit therapeutic interventions—as a potential reinforcement schedule for therapeutic effects.

The paper in this volume by Price and Fields seems to suggest that the "meaningfulness" of a placebo stimulus is a function of two variables, desire and expectancy, each of which can be measured quantitatively. I applaud Price and Fields for including the "desire" dimension, which has been very little studied previously and seems clinically fruitful. But I also resist any premature search for parsimony in the explanatory model. For one thing, their model is based only on placebo analgesia, and there is of course much more to the placebo effect than analgesia. More importantly, the narrative model of meaning suggests that the best way to discover the meaning that the patient attributes to an experience is to ask him or her about it, perhaps even explicitly asking the patient to tell the story that he or she has constructed to explain it. This implies in turn that we should consider using qualitative or ethnographic research methods in all studies of placebo effects where feasible. We may later be able to reduce the findings of these open-ended inquiries into meaning to visual analog scales or other methods which permit precise quantification; but we should be leery of using solely quantitative methods which seriously limit the subjects' range of allowed responses.

A Neurobiology of Meaning?

We may now turn to the question of what we can learn from studying the neural, immune, and biochemical pathways by which a stimulus that the person perceives as "meaningful" in a healing-related sense produces end-organ changes. I have argued that understanding this issue, by itself, will tell us only a part of the placebo story, unless we simultaneously study what stimuli the human organism regards as "meaningful" and why. And yet an understanding of this issue may cause us to see the question of meaningfulness in a new light, and perhaps also to see connections among disparate research findings that had previously seemed unrelated.

For example, current research into peptide receptors appears to be highly important for understanding the placebo response. It seems very likely that at least some placebo reactions are mediated by peptides; and the fact that brain cells, immune cells, and other body tissues all share receptors for these peptides hints at the outline of a psychosomatic information network which would allow us to make much more sense of placebo data than would any more simplistic, Cartesian-dualist model. Indeed, as Pert has argued, modern understanding of peptides knocks any Cartesian view of mind and body into a cocked hat. If identical peptide molecules are found to be active in the brain, the intestine, and the immune system, and cells in all three tissues have receptors for the same peptide, then it seems quite arbitrary to insist that a process goes on in the brain which is qualitatively different from processes which occur elsewhere in the body: "If you accept the premise that the mind is not just in the brain but that the mind is part of a communication network throughout the brain and body, then you can start to see how physiology can affect mental functioning on a moment-to-moment, hour-by-hour, day-by-day basis, much more than we give it credit for." (Moyers 1993, p. 181) And, we might add, we can start to see how the mind can affect physiological functioning on a moment-to-moment basis, as well.[4]

But it also turns out so far to be the case that these peptide receptors are thickly clustered in those parts of the brain functionally linked to emotions, and are seen least in the cerebral cortex and those centers normally associated with cognition. Does this situation mean that the placebo response is principally linked to the patient's emotional reaction to a healing encounter and that it effectively bypasses the patient's cognitive processes? Does it mean that there may be different biochemical pathways which link the cognitive centers of the brain to various end organ responses? Or does it mean that there is a closer link between emotion and cognition than we have previously tended to recognize—that in fact we humans come to know about the world in large part via our emotional reactions to what we perceive? Pert seems to favor the latter explanation: "One way to think of neuropeptides is that they direct energy. You can't do everything at every moment. Sometimes the energy needs to go toward digesting food. At other times more blood needs to flow through your spleen. If you've been challenged with a bug that can cause a fever, then you've got to put more energy into your spleen and less energy into digesting your food." (Moyers 1993, p. 181)

Pert illustrates this point by noting that angiotensin seems to be a water-conserving or water-seeking messenger at several levels. In the kidney and lung, it acts so as to minimize excretory water loss; applied to an animal brain, it appears to trigger an intense thirst reaction, even if the animal is actually overhydrated at the time. She refers to such a reaction as "emotion in the broadest sense." I take this to suggest that if a stimulus in our environment sets off processes that result in increased secretion of angiotensin within my body, then I will *feel thirsty*. If so, this is an emotion that is closely linked to cognitive processes, at least potentially. Possibly a person could feel thirsty, seek out something to drink, and not be consciously aware of this; but it seems at least as likely that a feeling of thirst will be accepted as information either about my internal state ("I didn't realize how long it had been since I drank that last soda") or about the outside world ("it must be a lot hotter out today than I realized"). And that information in turn will prompt further cognitive processing to discover reasons, possible solutions to a perceived problem, and so forth.

Pert is, in effect, claiming that the second major research agendum will inevitably influence the strategy of the first: "Thus, brain/drug receptors now form an experimentally accessible link between the classical scientific system of knowledge spanning the disciplines of psychology, ethology, and neuroanatomy and the more recently evolved system of knowledge encompassing biochemistry, immunology, and molecular biology. Chemical neuroanatomy has become an exciting level of inquiry into nervous system function as it brings behavior and molecules into the same hierarchy of knowledge." (Pert et al. 1985, p. 820s)

We should in passing praise Pert and colleagues for *not* arguing that the sciences of human behavior will ultimately be reduced to, or replaced by, peptide biochemistry, as some elements within modern U. S. psychiatry seem to be claiming. Their claim instead seems to be that if we wonder what it is that makes a certain social practice or personal encounter "meaningful" for an individual in the sense that it promotes healing, we might get some valuable clues by studying the distribution and function of neuropeptide receptors—even though in the end we will have to explain "meaningfulness" in psychological and sociocultural terms, and not merely in biochemical ones.

Conclusion

This discussion suggests that we should expand our vision of the two large placebo research agenda to include an important bit of inter-agenda business:

1. We should employ the psychological and social sciences to determine which circumstances of human social interaction alter the meaning of an illness experience for a given subject in a possible direction, thus setting a placebo response in motion. We should be ready to use conditioning theory as a part of this scientific effort, but without assuming that human cognition is unimportant. We should also be ready to expand our definition of cognitive processes to take into account the subject's emotional reaction to the situation as broadly defined (since emotions are experienced in the body in a way unlike how we experience mere ideas, and may thus provide important clues to the embodiment of cognition as well). We should employ qualitative and quantitative research strategies in a complementary fashion wherever feasible.

2. We should explore all physiological and biochemical pathways by which the brain "talks to" the body, to see which would best explain the specific end-organ changes that appear to be attributable to placebo responses.

3. We should be alert to clues from neurophysiology and neurochemistry which suggest that the human organism is especially well designed to react to particular environmental stimuli in particular ways. This information in turn may point to certain sorts of social stimuli which the individual is highly likely to perceive as "meaningful", or else to certain psychological states which are necessary precursors for the reception of a "meaningful stimulus." In turn, sociocultural investigations may suggest which sorts of stimuli are most important in various healing rituals or practices, and that information may provide neurobiologists with clues about which pathways or anatomic levels to look at.

Up until now, physicians have tended to be most sympathetic to the second research agendum in searching for an explanation or understanding of the placebo effect. (Recall the reaction in the medical press to the first reports of the placebo/naloxone connection in the 1970s, leading to confident reports that the placebo puzzle had finally been "solved" merely because one intermediate biochemical pathway had been proposed.) This is fully in keeping with the mind-body dualism or reductionism endemic in Western medical thinking. But it is not hard to see that for the clinician, the critical bit of research is rather the first agendum, so long as we wish to be powerful and persuasive healers. "Act so as to increase the secretion of neuropeptides which have receptors in the reticuloendothelial system" is hardly a very useful tip for the clinician; whereas, "Patients are much more likely to report later relief of symptoms when they feel fully listened to when they first come to you with their problem" gives very practical, how-to advice for those of us who would wish, in our own humble way, to emulate Shaw's B. B.

A final question requires some degree of clairvoyance into the future success of the various research agenda. Is "placebo effect" destined to be a disappearing category? As we develop better understanding of which sorts of behavioral cues alter a person's meaning, and which psychosomatic pathways are activated as a result, will we not develop a much more precise nosology for the phenomena which "placebo effect" now covers as a wastebasket term?

I would suggest that a lot will depend upon whether both the most satisfying behavioral theory and the most satisfying account of the bodily pathways turn out to be unified or multiple. That is, will we end up explaining "meaningfulness" by a single cluster of closely associated psychosocial stimuli; or will a multiplicity of stimuli turn out to be implicated, with some operating for some people in some situations, and others in others? And will we end up, as now appears to be the case, postulating multiple psychosomatic pathways by which placebos may operate (for example, endorphin, catecholamine, and neuroimmune); or will we come to see that the apparent multiplicity can be better explained by a single unified hypothesis (for example, a small number of neuropeptides which share receptors in the brain, pituitary, and immune system)?

I can imagine several scenarios that would be compatible with retaining "placebo effect" as our overarching concept. This view would obviously make sense if the behavioral:physiological relationship turned out to be either one:one or one:many. It would also make the most sense in one sort of many:many scenario, that is, where (for example) we could identify behavioral "meaningfulness" stimuli A, B, and C; and physiological pathways X, Y, and Z; but there was no predictable relationship between any one behavioral stimulus and any one pathway. That is, in one situation, A might trigger a placebo response by activating the X pathway, while in another situation it might do so by activating the Z pathway.

The only scenario compatible with a disappearance of the term "placebo effect" from our lexicon would seem to be a many:many relationship but with a high degree of correlation between one behavioral stimulus and one bodily pathway. In our preceding example, that would mean that behavioral stimulus A always operated by activating the X pathway, B by activating Y, and C by activating Z. We might then replace imprecise talk of "placebo effects" by speaking instead, say, of "alpha effects," "beta effects," and "gamma effects" to label the end results of the $A{\rightarrow}X$, $B{\rightarrow}Y$, and $C{\rightarrow}Z$ processes, respectively. This example would be especially attractive if the processes explained the relief of different symptoms or different diseases—for instance, if the $A{\to}X$ process turned out to account for all of what we now call "placebo effects" in rheumatoid arthritis, whereas the $B{\to}Y$ process accounted for all placebo effects previously observed in respiratory infections. It seems quite premature, to me, to predict whether something like this scenario is likely to come about. Thus, at least for the foreseeable future, "placebo effect" seems a useful label for an important body of multidisciplinary and interdisciplinary research.

We would like, in the end, to tell physicians how to act more like B. B. But we don't wish to reconstruct the authoritarian and paternalistic world of medicine in which B. B. played a role at the turn of the century. While the occasional patient will be too ill, too frightened, or too overwhelmed to do more than submit to the physician's soothing care, we do not want physicians to use those extreme instances to justify depriving the average patient of the right to participate in medical decisions to whatever extent the patient wishes. We would like our modern B. B.'s not only to have substantial powers to vanquish illness but also to possess the humility to use that power only in responsible ways (Brody 1992). The proper dose of humility may be provided by a recent observation by Bulger (1990), that the patient, and not the physician, is in the end the therapeutic agent—the placebo stimulus, whether the physician's behavior or something else, simply uncorks the internal pharmacopeia which all humans possess as a biologically programmed tool for self-healing.

References

Brody, H. 1980. *Placebos and the Philosophy of Medicine.* Chicago: University of Chicago Press.

———. 1982. "The Lie That Heals: The Ethics of Giving Placebos." *Annals of Internal Medicine,* 97:112–118.

———. 1985. "Placebo Effect: An Examination of Grunbaum's Definition." In *Placebo: Theory, Research, and Mechanisms.* In L. White, B. Tursky, and G. E. Schwartz. New York: Guilford Press.

———. 1986. "The Placebo Response. Part I: Exploring the Myths. Part II: Use in Clinical Practice." *Drug Therapy,* 16(7):106–131.

———. 1992. *The Healer's Power.* New Haven: Yale University Press.

———. 1995. "Placebo." In *Encyclopedia of Bioethics,* 2nd ed. W. T. Reich., ed. New York: Macmillan.

Bruner, J. 1986. *Actual Minds, Possible Worlds.* Cambridge, Mass.: Harvard University Press.

Bulger, R. J. 1990. "The Demise of the Placebo Effect in the Practice of Scientific Medicine—A Natural Progression or an Undesirable Aberration?" *Transactions of the American Clinical and Climatological Association,* 102:285–293.

Engel, G. 1987. "How Long Must Medicine's Science Be Bound by a Seventeenth Century World View?" In K. L. White, ed., *Dialogue at Wickenburg.* Menlo Park, Calif.: Henry J. Kaiser Family Foundation.

Findley, T. 1953. "The Placebo and the Physician." *Medical Clinics of North America,* 37:1821–1826.

Houston, W. R. 1938. "The Doctor Himself as a Therapeutic Agent." *Annals of Internal Medicine,* 11:1416–1425.

Kleinman, A. M., and L. H. Sung. 1976. "Why Do Indigenous Healers Successfully Heal?" Paper presented at a workshop, "The Healing Process," Michigan State University, East Lansing, April.

Moyers, B. 1993. *Healing and the Mind.* New York: Doubleday.

Novack, D. H. 1987. "Therapeutic Aspects of the Clinical Encounter." *Journal of General Internal Medicine,* 2:346–355.

Pert, C. B., M. R. Ruff, R. J. Weber, and M. Herkenham. 1985. "Neuropeptides and Their Receptors: A Psychosomatic Network." *Journal of Immunology,* 135(supplement):820s–826s.

Notes

1. Irving Kirsch made this point very effectively at the conference.
2. See Robert Hahn's paper in this collection for a quite different account of the nocebo effect. I do not share Hahn's view, discussed at the conference, that the pathways which we commonly associate with placebo effects today seem incapable of explaining nocebo effects, since many of these pathways have modulatory properties which could account for either returning a disordered process back toward homeostasis, or else exacerbating it further, depending on the timing and direction of the modulatory mechanism.
3. I am grateful to Gordon Kaufman and Stephen Kosslyn for helpful discussion of these points at the conference, and to Anne Harrington for helpful suggestions in clarifying this portion of the manuscript.
4. The heuristic appeal of these findings as a new and expanded way of understanding the "embodiedness" of the mind depends on Pert's assertion that neuropeptide molecules travel freely between the brain and peripheral

sites. Otherwise, the fact that the same small molecule is used as a biologic signal at two separate bodily sites is merely another example of the genetic parsimony of biological systems. John Dowling, at the conference, has informed me that there are reasons to doubt the easy passage of these molecules in and out of the brain, which appears consistent with the medical concept of the "blood-brain barrier"; I lack the expertise to resolve this issue.

Toward a Neurobiology of Placebo Analgesia

5

Howard L. Fields
Donald D. Price

Introduction

Placebo responses are an object of continuing fascination for a broad range of people in academic and clinical settings. Such fascination derives, in no small part, from the seeming improbability of mental processes exerting influence over physical events such as disease. Implicit to this presumed improbability is the assumption that subjective awareness (that is, the conscious mind) and physical phenomena are ontologically distinct. Under this paradigm, it is, naturally, difficult to envision how subjective awareness might affect the physical state of the body.

This mind-body dualism is popular partly because it arises out of common experience. It is clear, however, that this common dualistic view neglects the central role played by the brain. The brain's role has been obscure because although an individual's conscious experience of both the body and the external world is produced by the activity of the brain, brain activity per se is imperceptible to oneself. The individual has no experience of the agency of the brain but is aware of an apparent subject (the conscious mind) and apparent objects (parts of the body and the external world), and thus the dualistic belief is created that everything is subject or object. It is not surprising, given the universality of this experience, that mind-body dualism is pervasive in both popular philosophy and medical practice.

It is not the purpose of this chapter to discuss the logical shortcomings of mind-body dualism. Suffice it to say that this dualism is at best

93

an incomplete view and one that engenders unnecessary confusion about such phenomena as placebo responses. If, however, one recognizes that brain activity both regulates bodily function and generates conscious experience, much of the confusion about the bodily effects of subjective experience is dispelled. This approach, which we might call a neuralist view, obviates the mind-body mechanism problem because it treats subjective phenomena (the conscious mind) as products of nervous system activity.

Neural Representations

Both observable behaviors and subjective experience are created by functional networks of neurons in the brain. The activity of such networks at a given time has meaning that is based on its correlation with nonneural entities such as physical stimuli, memories, ideas, and feelings. The active network is said to represent these things. A neural representation has three critical aspects: it is an objective physical entity; it is an active representation of something else (for example, an object, an image, the self); and it is the generator of subjective experience. Neural representations can create a nexus between subjective experience and the physical (objective) world. This neuralist approach avoids the problem of how a subjective "mind" could act on the objective and physical body. The issue of whether and how the subjective "mind" could produce changes in neural activity, although potentially critical to the issue of placebo mechanisms, is beyond the scope of this chapter.

How might placebo analgesia be understood within this neuralist framework? If a person's body undergoes a tissue destructive process (for example, a myocardial infarction), activation of tissue sensory neurons by this process will induce in the central nervous system a pattern of neural activity (representation) that gives rise to the subjective experience of pain. Administration of an analgesic such as morphine will alter that representation in a way that reduces pain. Administration of a placebo can also alter the neural representation induced by a tissue destructive process. The placebo response of an individual can be thought of as resulting from an interaction between the neural representation induced by the experience of receiving a placebo and the representation induced by the process being treated (for instance, painful tissue damage). In addition, an individual's memories, the environmental context, and specific sensory stimuli all contribute to an ensemble of interacting neural representations. This ensemble generates a subjective experience and can concomitantly act on the body through physical (not metaphysical or magical) channels. Furthermore, the ensemble could in theory be viewed with functional imaging—for example, positron emission tomography (PET)—but such an observation would only confirm what we already know: that there has been an objective change in that part of the physical body called the brain.

Neurobiology Is a Useful Approach to the Understanding of Placebo Mechanisms

If one accepts the causal relationship of the nervous system to subjective awareness, it follows that study of the nervous system is critical to formulating a mechanistic explanation of placebo responses. To this end, a reassessment of the issue of placebo mechanisms is timely. In the past three decades, enormous progress has been made in understanding many relevant aspects of the function of the nervous system. Our analytical tools have brought us close to explaining such phenomena as vision, movement, and learning at the level of neural connections and activity. In this chapter, we will address the issue of whether we are at the point of exploiting our improved understanding of the brain better to comprehend placebo administration's therapeutic effects. We will focus on placebo analgesia. First we will describe how placebo responses are studied, and then we will describe those of its components that lend themselves to explanation at the level of neural mechanisms and will propose testable hypotheses for those components. Finally, we will briefly summarize current knowledge about central nervous system pain modulating circuits and discuss evidence supporting the hypothesis that these circuits contribute to placebo analgesia.

Why Study Pain Relief?

The study of analgesia offers an excellent opportunity to understand placebo responses at the level of neural mechanisms. Robust placebo analgesic effects have been demonstrated across a variety of experimental and clinical situations (Liberman 1964; Levine and Gordon 1984;

Grevert et al. 1983a; Gracely et al. 1983). Though pain is subjective, it is a ubiquitous human experience and clinical problem. Furthermore, since it can be elicited by quantifiable stimuli, the psychophysics of pain assessment is well developed (Price 1988). The same stimuli that elicit human pain produce aversive behaviors in animals and activate well-known central nervous system pathways. Since these pathways are homologous across mammalian species, including humans, results obtained in animal studies are likely relevant to human experiences of pain. Importantly, brain circuitry which selectively modulates pain transmission has been discovered. Such circuitry offers a potential substrate for the generation of placebo analgesia. Furthermore, the discovery of neurotransmitters (such as endogenous opioids) that are involved in pain modulation offers an opportunity pharmacologically to enhance or block placebo analgesia. In this way, hypotheses about the neural mechanism of placebo can be tested in both laboratory animals and human subjects. A similar approach could be taken to address the neural mechanisms of other placebo actions.

Detailed and useful definitions of the placebo have been presented elsewhere and will not be reviewed here (see chapters by Grunbaum and Brody in White et al. 1985). However, some definitions are in order. The reduction in pain in an individual caused by placebo administration will be called the *analgesic placebo response*. The *placebo analgesic effect* will be defined as the mean placebo-produced reduction in pain in a group of subjects.

Confounding Factors in the Study of Analgesic Placebo Responses

Before we address the neural mechanism of placebo analgesia, we must describe the phenomenon itself. Unfortunately, there are two critical technical problems limiting our ability to describe it. First, because pain is a subjective experience, it cannot be directly observed (except when it occurs in oneself). In order to investigate rigorously the phenomenon of placebo analgesia, it is necessary to limit bias in self-observation and reporting of pain. The difficulties of establishing a rigorously double-blind experiment are well known and have been discussed extensively both in this volume (Kirsch) and elsewhere (Ross and Buckalew 1985; Max et al. 1991).

Secondly, "spontaneous" variation in pain level in the absence of any treatment is common and confounds the study of placebo responses. Any treatment manipulation may be followed by a reduction in pain level, simply by chance. To attribute the drop in pain to any antecedent treatment, including placebo, is therefore an inference. The validity of that inference depends on the uncertain (and often erroneous) assumption that, had the placebo not been given, the post-placebo pain level at a given point in time would have been higher than the level that was actually observed. Such an assumption may be tested by making multiple observations of untreated subjects to determine the range, mean, and variance of their pain, giving us baseline information—a "natural history" of pain. It should be pointed out that withholding treatment for pain in clinical practice is hardly more "natural" than treating it and could introduce a new source of variability. Nonetheless, an untreated control group is an important part of any experimental approach to studying the placebo analgesic response.

Because few studies of the placebo analgesic effect have included an untreated comparison group, we have very little knowledge of the effect's magnitude, time course, or frequency of occurrence. In fact, in the absence of a no-treatment group, it is usually difficult to know whether placebo administration has produced any effect at all.

The Difficulty of Observing Individual Placebo

Although an increasing number of workers in the field now understand the natural history issue, overlooking the importance of an untreated comparison group remains a major source of confusion in current literature on placebo (Wall 1994; Wickramasekera 1985). This situation results in the frequently unwarranted conclusion that a placebo responder can be identified (or that an analgesic placebo response has occurred) if a subject's pain is observed to decrease following placebo treatment. As an example of this mistake, consider the problem of episodic migraine headache. Most migraine sufferers have intermittent headaches. They have two- to three-day episodes of severe pain, separated by days to weeks of no pain. Untreated, the pain rises from none to severe and falls to none again. The duration of the attack is limited by unknown and unpredictable mechanisms. Therefore, episodes of headache in the same individual vary in their severity and duration. Since the pain of an attack is self-limited, any treatment (or no treatment) given during the attack will be followed, after a variable interval, by relief. If a placebo were given during an attack, relief would certainly follow; however, for that attack, we would have no way to know whether placebo administration changed the time course of the headache pain.

This example reveals the inferential (as opposed to observational) nature of an individual occurrence of the analgesic placebo response (or, for that matter, any treatment response). In most clinical situations, the observed time course of pain intensity in an individual yields only tentative and partial information about the occurrence of a placebo response. Because we do not know what would have happened had we not given the placebo, we cannot attribute any subsequent relief to the administration of the placebo. In fact, for an individual treatment, it may be impossible to know whether the placebo relieved or worsened pain. To illustrate this point, consider the following two thought experiments.

In the first experiment, the time course of pain in the absence of treatment is one of steady decline during the observation period (thick line, Figure 5.1, upper graph). In this experiment, the effect of giving the placebo (the treatment) is an increment of pain (interrupted line, top of Figure 5.1). Although the treatment has worsened the pain, the net effect is a decline in pain level. In this extreme case, although the effect of placebo administration was increased pain, the placebo manipulation was followed by relief. Increase in pain following placebo (or sham treatment) is sometimes called the nocebo effect.

Now we consider the opposing situation. The natural history here is a steady rise in pain intensity over the observation period (thick line, Figure 5.1, lower graph). In this situation, the placebo causes a decrement in pain. Despite the decrement, the sum of placebo effect and natural history is a rise in pain. In this case, although the placebo produced a reduction in pain, the patient's net pain continued to increase. Were we unaware of the natural history, we would have erroneously concluded that the placebo had had no effect or had worsened the pain.

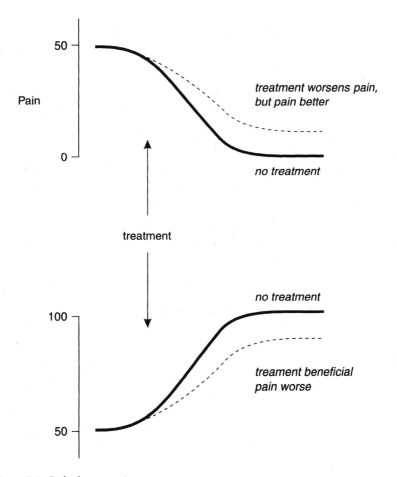

Figure 5.1 Gedanken experiment

These thought experiments demonstrate that, because of variability in the magnitude and time course of pain intensity in clinical situations, group comparisons are usually the only reliable way to study the phenomenon of placebo analgesia.

An individual occurrence of placebo analgesic effect could be defined by comparing the individual's postplacebo pain level at a given time with a group-derived mean. If the individual response was significantly below the group mean, one could conclude (at a defined level of confidence) that a response to the placebo had occurred (see Liberman

1964). Alternately, one might administer placebo to an individual for an episodic painful condition and then compare the mean pain level with that for multiple untreated occurrences of the same condition in the same individual. The latter approach, however, has both practical and theoretical problems. It makes the patient into an experimental subject, causing additional discomfort and stress, and it could change the natural history of the patient's pain.

The Phenomenology of Placebo Analgesia

Despite the uncertainty surrounding individual response, the placebo analgesic effect is a robust phenomenon. Several investigators have reported a significant placebo analgesic effect compared with an untreated control group (Gelfand et al. 1963; Liberman 1964; Levine and Gordon 1984; Gracely et al. 1983; Grevert et al. 1983a).

Liberman (1964) showed that placebo administration can, in labor and postpartum pain, produce a mean shift of one level on a category intensity scale (for example, from severe to moderate). Using experimental ischemic arm pain, Grevert et al. (1983a) showed a mean placebo effect of about 1 cm on a 10 cm visual analog intensity scale. Although Levine et al. (1981) found a similar mean magnitude of placebo effect in dental postoperative pain, their data suggested that individual analgesic placebo responses might actually be severalfold larger than the mean but occur only in a minority of individuals. Levine et al. (1981) also compared open administration of placebo to hidden infusion of morphine. Placebo was found to be equivalent to about 5 mg of intravenous morphine. Importantly, their data suggested that, when it occurs, the analgesic response of an individual to either morphine or placebo is similar in magnitude (about 5 cm on the 10 cm visual analog scale), but that the probability of an analgesic response to morphine increases as the morphine dose increases.

What Aspects of Placebo Analgesia Can Be Explained at the Level of Neural Mechanisms?

When a placebo analgesic effect has been demonstrated, it is appropriate then to explore what has occurred in the central nervous system to produce the observed reduction in pain.

There are formidable problems confronting those who would attempt to study the neural mechanisms underlying any human behavior, especially subjective experiences such as placebo analgesic effects. Although technically possible, it is neither ethical nor currently feasible to carry out in human subjects the invasive anatomical and physiological experiments needed to study the relevant neural circuits at the required level of spatial and temporal resolution. On the other hand, data obtained from animal studies may not generalize to even superficially similar human behaviors. In fact, certain complex human experiences, such as those related to culture and language, probably have no animal equivalent. Although the placebo response may depend critically upon such cognitive factors (see Chapter 6), we do not understand their role at the level of neural mechanisms. Nonetheless, neural mechanisms of some aspects of the placebo response can be approached, and we now turn our focus to these aspects.

Three currently active areas of study in neurobiology are relevant to placebo analgesia: learning and memory, threat-elicited defensive behaviors, and pain modulation. Threat and pain modulation are linked during the production of conditioned fear (Helmstetter and Tershner 1994; Fanselow 1984, 1991). There is growing knowledge of the circuitry underlying several types of learning and memory, conditioned defensive reactions, and pain modulation. We may thus consider three issues in the development of a neural hypothesis of placebo analgesia. First, what associations are relevant to the placebo effect—that is, what triggers it? Secondly, what is the contribution of conditioned defensive behavior to its production? And finally, once triggered, how is the analgesic effect produced?

Learning Analgesia

The evidence reviewed in other chapters of this volume (see Chapters 6 and 8) establishes that associative learning is, or can be, a major contributor to placebo analgesia.

The triggering process for analgesia requires that the subject identify environmental cues that are linked to the placebo manipulation and are associated with pain relief. The environmental stimuli may be visual (the doctor's white coat), auditory (the nurse's voice), olfactory (the smell of disinfectant), or tactile (the prick of a needle). In some cases, the physical properties of the relevant stimuli might be directly associated with relief. In other cases, it is the symbolic content of the stimuli that is associated with relief. In either case, stimuli effective for producing analgesia have acquired meaning through previous learning.

For example, the phrase, "this is a powerful pain killer," has symbolic meaning independent of the (auditory) modality used to communicate it. The message could, with equal effectiveness, be presented visually (via a note or sign language) or through touch (via Braille). It is the symbolic content of the message that actually produces the expectation of relief and triggers analgesia. Acts of treatment include both a direct sensory experience and a potentially complex symbolic communication. A subject can learn to associate both elements with pain relief, and either or both may contribute to the analgesic response. The contribution of a symbolic communication, whose meaning is unique to human individual and cultural experience, currently cannot be studied at the level of neural mechanisms. On the other hand, to the extent that an analgesic response is triggered by simple sensory cues, it can be modeled in animals and its neural mechanisms studied using conventional neurobiological methods. In fact, there is evidence that sensory cues can make an important contribution to the placebo analgesic effect.

Three important studies demonstrate the contribution of conditioning to placebo analgesia. Laska and Sunshine (1973) examined the effect of prior drug administration on the magnitude of placebo analgesia. Hospitalized patients with a variety of acutely painful conditions (fractures, postoperative pain, and so on) were placed in groups that received identical tablets containing either placebo or varying doses of an active analgesic (propoxyphene) as a first treatment. Twenty-four hours later, all patients who needed pain medication were given placebo tablets. The mean analgesic effect of the placebo was significantly correlated with the dose of propoxyphene given as the first treatment. This result isolates some dose-related drug effect, most likely pain relief, as an independent variable that can contribute to the analgesic effectiveness of a subsequent, similar-appearing placebo. This is a conditioning paradigm that can easily be modeled in animals.

Voudouris et al. (1990) used a fake treatment to demonstrate the contribution to placebo effect of associations between reduced pain and other environmental cues. In conditioning trials, they put a cream on the skin and, by reducing the intensity of an applied electrical stimulus, led subjects to believe that the cream was an anesthetic. In subsequent trials of electrical stimulation through the cream, those conditioned by reduced stimulus intensity reported less pain compared with untrained subjects. Clearly, the contingent pairing of reduced pain with other environmental cues can lead to a conditioned analgesic effect.

If classical conditioning is a major factor in the production of placebo analgesia, repeated administration of a placebo should lead to extinction of its analgesic effect. This prediction was confirmed by Fedele et al. (1989), who randomly assigned women with dysmenor-rhea to placebo or nonsteroidal anti-inflammatory drug treatment. Patients were given three days of either treatment over four successive menstrual cycles. The placebo was as effective as the active drug for the first cycle, but by the fourth cycle, placebo efficacy had dropped by about 90 percent. Clearly, whatever contribution was made by cognitive and symbolic processing, repeated administration of inactive tablets (loss of drug effect) was sufficient to abolish placebo analgesia.

These studies indicate that when effective drugs are paired with a variety of neutral environmental stimuli, the environmental stimuli (for example, a tablet's shape and color) acquire analgesic potency. This type of conditioning contributes to the placebo component of both active and inactive treatments and can be modeled in animals.

Conditioned Analgesia in Animals

Conditioned analgesic responses in animals are robust and may be elicited in ways that suggest relevance to human placebo analgesia. The most extensively studied form of conditioned analgesia is seen in fear-evoked defense responses. In the typical experiment, rats are subjected to an inescapable noxious stimulus, leading to stress and apparent analgesia (Watkins and Mayer 1982; Watkins et al. 1983; Fanselow 1984, 1991; Helmstetter and Tershner 1994). Animals recover pain sensitivity, but when they are later returned to the apparatus in which the noxious stimulus was administered, the context is sufficient to produce an analgesic effect.

Analgesia associated with conditioned fear can be blocked by the opioid antagonist naloxone or by lesions of a specific neural circuit implicated in the elaboration of defense behaviors to threat (Helmstetter and Tershner 1994; also see later). Although fear is frequently observed in the paradigms used to produce conditioned analgesia, fear may not be an essential mediator of subsequent context-elicited analgesia (Kinscheck et al. 1984). This type of conditioned analgesia has been proposed as a model for placebo analgesia (Watkins and Mayer 1982).

Analgesia can also be classically conditioned in animals by pairing opioid administration with a neutral taste cue (Miller et al. 1990). Interestingly, this form of classically conditioned analgesia can be attenuated by the opioid antagonist naloxone. These animal studies demonstrate that analgesia can be learned and indicate that specific circuitry and neurotransmitters can contribute to this effect.

Fear, Anxiety, and Human Placebo Analgesia

Because specific central nervous system circuitry has been implicated in analgesia associated with conditioned fear in animal models, the contribution, if any, of fear and anxiety to human placebo analgesia has theoretical importance in the quest to elucidate its neural mechanism. Unfortunately, the relationship of anxiety to human placebo analgesia is complex. There is limited evidence suggesting that placebo analgesia is greater in situations producing greater anxiety. Some experimenters, for example, have suggested that clinical pains are more susceptible to placebo than experimental pains, and there is some evidence that more severe pains are more likely to be relieved by placebo (Beecher 1956; Levine et al. 1979). However, the interpretation of these findings is complicated by the fact that anxiety or "stress" is sufficient to produce an opioid-mediated analgesic response in humans without placebo administration (Gracely et al. 1983; Pitman et al. 1990; Willer et al. 1981; Schull et al. 1981). Furthermore, the anxiolytic diazepam reduces the analgesic effect of stress (Willer and Ernst 1986). These studies suggest that there are circumstances in which relief of anxiety can be associated with a reduction of analgesia.

Despite these observations, the view that placebo administration relieves pain by reducing anxiety is commonplace and is supported by some experimental evidence (Evans 1985, in White). In theory, placebo administration could have two opposing actions: to produce analgesia and to reduce stress-induced analgesia. One possible explanation for this apparent paradox is that although the placebo may reduce anxiety after it is given, the presence of stress/anxiety prior to treatment increases the likelihood or magnitude of the placebo analgesic effect. Such a possibility is consistent with our proposal that desire for relief is a critical variable both in placebo analgesia and in pain-related anxiety (see Chapter 6). This is clearly an important topic for future study.

Pain-Modulating Circuitry

The discovery of brain circuits selective for pain modulation was a major conceptual advance in understanding placebo analgesic responses. Although there are probably multiple pain-modulating circuits, we best know those that selectively modulate pain transmission pathways at their origin in the spinal cord. The most extensively studied of these pathways includes interconnected neurons in the brainstem (midbrain periaqueductal gray, or PAG, and its vicinity, and the rostral ventral medulla, or RVM). Output neurons of this brainstem circuit (in the RVM) are directly connected to pain relay neurons in the spinal cord. Stimulation of this brainstem circuit inhibits pain transmission pathways (Figure 5.2).

The same brainstem-to-spinal-cord circuit contributes to the effect of narcotic analgesics such as morphine. Many neurons in PAG and RVM have opiate receptors (Delfs et al. 1994; Atweh and Kuhar 1977). These sites are densely innervated by neurons containing endogenous opioid peptides (Basbaum and Fields 1984; Fields et al. 1991). Minute amounts of opioids injected into RVM or PAG produce analgesia (Yaksh 1988), which is potentiated by a fear-inducing context (Lea et al. 1994).

We have quite detailed knowledge of the neural mechanisms by which opioids act at some of these sites to produce behavioral analgesia (see Fields et al. 1991 for review). For example, there are two classes

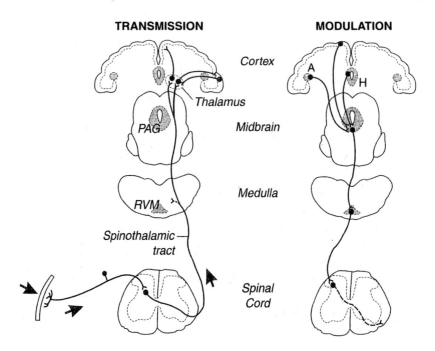

Figure 5.2 Transmission and modulation in pain transmission pathways

of pain-modulating neurons (Figure 5.3) in the RVM. One class, the on cell, becomes active just prior to withdrawal from a noxious stimulus. This cell class is directly inhibited by endogenous opioids and appears to have a facilitatory effect on pain. A second class of RVM neuron, the off cell, pauses just before a withdrawal reflex. Off cells are not directly affected by opioids; however, they are inhibited by on cells. Following opioid inhibition of the on cell, off cells increase their activity. Off cells appear to have an inhibitory effect on pain transmission. Figure 5.4 shows a diagram of these connections.

There is direct evidence that the pain-modulating circuitry just described can play a key role in conditioned analgesia. Thus lesions of or microinjection of an opioid antagonist drug into the PAG or RVM can block some forms of conditioned analgesia (Helmstetter and Tershner 1994; Kim et al. 1993; Watkins and Mayer 1982). Although this pain-modulating network does not explain the conditioning process, it contributes to the resultant analgesia.

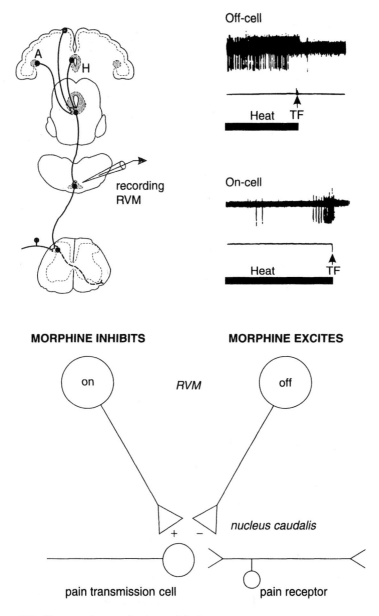

Off-cell

Heat   TF

On-cell

Heat   TF

MORPHINE INHIBITS   **MORPHINE EXCITES**

on   *RVM*   off

nucleus caudalis

pain transmission cell   pain receptor

Figure 5.3 The two classes of pain-modulating neurons

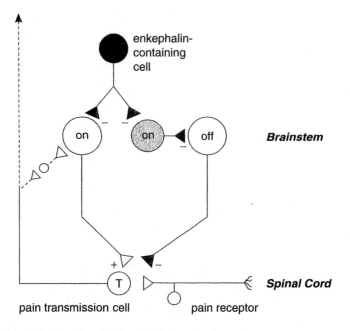

Figure 5.4 Opioid-mediated pain modulating circuit

If this circuitry does mediate some forms of conditioned analgesia in animals and if similar processes occur in humans, it is possible that circuitry homologous to that mediating conditioned analgesia in animals contributes to human placebo analgesia. Although speculative at this point, the hypothesis is potentially testable.

Does Placebo Analgesia in Humans Involve Opioid-Mediated Pain-Modulating Circuitry?

Since it is very difficult to test directly a specific neural circuit hypothesis underlying a complex human behavior, we must primarily rely upon indirect evidence. At present, we can only establish whether our hypothesis is reasonable and propose experiments to further test it.

For our hypothesis to be correct, humans must have the pain-modulating circuitry elucidated in those species that have been experimentally studied. There are several independent lines of evidence supporting this idea. The brainstem-to-spinal-cord circuitry implicated in conditioned analgesia is highly conserved in a variety of mammalian species, including rodents, carnivores, primates, and marsupials. Importantly, the distribution of neurotransmitters, including opioid peptides, in this pathway also appears to be similar in a number of species, including humans (Emson et al. 1984; Pittius et al. 1984). The homogeneity of pain-modulating circuitry across this diversity of species leaves little doubt that such circuitry is present in humans. Furthermore, opioid drugs that relieve clinically significant pain in patients are effective in inhibiting escape behaviors in all tested mammalian species. In animals, this analgesic effect is exerted in part through actions upon the brain-stem-to-spinal cord circuitry that mediates conditioned analgesia. Finally, the idea that homologous circuitry can produce analgesia in humans is strongly supported by the remarkable observation that patients with chronic pain report relief during stimulation of specific sites in the human midbrain. Although these brain stimulation studies have not been rigorous, similar results have been reported by many surgical groups (Baskin et al. 1986; Boivie and Meyerson 1982). The effect is selective for pain and is elicited only by stimulating midbrain regions homologous to those that inhibit behavioral and neural responses to noxious stimuli in rats, cats, and primates. This observation in humans represents a critical extension of animal work, because it indicates that the reduced behavioral response to noxious stimuli produced by midbrain stimulation is accompanied by subjective pain relief.

In summary, several independent lines of evidence support the assumption that humans have neural circuitry homologous to that which mediates conditioned analgesia and contributes to opioid analgesia in animals.

Is there any evidence that this opioid-mediated pain-modulating circuit can be activated under physiological conditions in humans? Work using the opioid antagonist naloxone to enhance pain yields an affirmative answer. We may reason as follows: There are endogenous opioid peptides and opioid receptors at central nervous system sites implicated in pain modulation. Exogenous opioids, which are potent pain relievers in humans, presumably act at the same receptor sites as the endogenous opioids. If these assumptions are true, there should be circumstances under which endogenous opioids reduce pain, and under such circumstances administration of an opioid antagonist should block pain reduction.

Levine et al. (1978a) were the first to demonstrate clearly that, when compared with placebo, 10 mg of naloxone significantly worsens postoperative pain. Naloxone is an excellent drug to use in studies of subjective phenomena because, at the doses used in these studies, it is virtually nonpsychoactive in opioid-naive, pain-free subjects (Grevert et al. 1978, 1983b; Wolkowitz and Tinklenberg 1985). Because naloxone produces no subjective effect that could consistently betray its administration, it can be given in a true double-blind manipulation. Naloxone hyperalgesia has been replicated in studies using both clinical and experimental pains (see Grevert and Goldstein 1985, for a review).

The significance of these naloxone studies is twofold. First, they demonstrate, under controlled conditions, that an endogenous pain-modulating system in humans can be reproducibly activated. Second, the hyperalgesic response to naloxone suggests that the pain-modulating system has opioid links. One obvious possibility is that it is the same pain-modulating network just described.

We now come to the final issue in our discussion: is there evidence that placebo analgesia is produced through the action of an opioid-mediated pain-modulating circuit?

Several studies have addressed this question. In the first study (Levine et al. 1978b), dental postoperative pain patients were given a placebo and then randomized to receive either a second placebo or naloxone. Since the typical natural history of pain under these conditions is a steady increase for up to five hours (Levine et al. 1979), those patients whose pain increased following the first placebo were labeled placebo nonresponders; those whose pain decreased or did not change were called responders. Naloxone increased pain in placebo responders but had no effect on nonresponders. A subsequent study (Levine and Gordon 1984) used identical methods but included a natural history group that received hidden infusions of either naloxone or vehicle. In the later study, naloxone had no effect upon patients that had had no overt treatment. Together, these studies demonstrate that placebo analgesia can be significantly reduced by naloxone.

Studies by Grevert et al. (1983a) support this conclusion. Using tourniquet ischemic pain as a model, they demonstrated a significant placebo analgesic effect. Whereas naloxone (10 mg) did not affect pain in the control group (who had not been given a placebo), it did significantly reduce placebo analgesia.

A separate line of evidence implicates opioids in placebo analgesia. Lipman et al. (1990) reported endogenous opioidlike material in the cerebrospinal fluid of chronic pain patients whose pain level dropped following placebo administration.

Although an opioid contribution to placebo analgesia appears to be established, it is important to point out that placebo analgesia, under some circumstances, may have a nonopioid component (Grevert et al. 1983a). And as mentioned previously, stress can elicit an opioid-mediated analgesic effect in the absence of placebo administration. For example, Gracely et al. (1983), using the dental postoperative pain model and both open and hidden naloxone infusions, demonstrated that 10 mg naloxone can produce hyperalgesia without overt placebo administration. They concluded that placebo administration was not necessary to elicit opioid-mediated analgesia. Interestingly, in contrast to the method of Levine et al. (1978b, 1979, 1984), subjects in the Gracely et al. study were not given nitrous oxide or diazepam for their surgery, so that pain and anxiety levels during and after the procedure were probably higher than in the Levine studies.

These studies strongly suggest that there are circumstances under which human analgesic responses with a significant endogenous opioid component can occur. One such circumstance is administration of placebo to a subject in pain. Although by no means conclusive, these data provide an evidentiary link between the behavioral phenomenon of placebo analgesia in humans and specific pain-modulating circuitry, and they are consistent with the hypothesis that the therapeutic act can trigger pain-modulating circuitry with opioid links. Such circuitry appears to be present in the human central nervous system, and its rodent homologue is well-described.

Conclusion

Placebo analgesia is a robust phenomenon that can be demonstrated in clinical and experimental settings. Classical conditioning plays a demonstrable role in determining its mean magnitude. Anxiety may be a contributing factor. In rodents, analgesia can be classically conditioned and is mediated by a central nervous system pain-modulating circuit with opioid links. Humans appear to possess homologous opioid-mediated circuitry. Under defined circumstances, placebo analgesia in humans is naloxone-reversible. We propose that placebo analgesia in humans is produced in part through circuitry homologous to that underlying conditioned analgesia in rodents.

At the same time, the study of placebo analgesia is in its early stages. We still have little information about the time course and magnitude of placebo analgesia in different types of pain. We also lack detailed information on environmental cues that trigger or enhance it. In light of the recent progress toward elucidating the neurotransmitters involved in pain modulation, renewed investigation of the pharmacology of placebo analgesia is especially timely. It will be important to determine the circumstances in which endogenous opioids do or do not contribute to placebo analgesia. The role of nonopioid neurotransmitter systems (for example, serotonin and norepinephrine) can also be usefully investigated.

Although there are limitations to investigating hypotheses about pain-modulating circuitry in the human nervous system, several methodologies that are currently available could potentially elucidate the neural mechanisms of placebo. These include single neuron recordings in the human somatosensory thalamus, functional imaging methods, such as positron emission tomography (PET), single photon emission computed tomography, and functional magnetic resonance imaging. PET has already successfully demonstrated brain activity elicited by noxious stimuli (Casey et al. 1994). In theory, this methodology could test circuit hypotheses by studying subjects before and after placebo administration and comparing them with untreated controls. Less sophisticated means can be used as well: indirect correlates of pain, such as autonomic parameters, withdrawal reflexes, and plasma "stress" hormone levels can objectively measure placebo responses. For example, the R-III is a spinally mediated withdrawal reflex that can be noninvasively measured in human subjects, and it correlates well with reported pain intensity. Inhibition of this reflex during placebo analgesia would support the hypothesis that a brainstem spinal pathway was involved. Improved knowledge of the phenomenology of placebo analgesia, pain-modulating neural circuits and their pharmacology, and improved resolution of functional imaging techniques should lead to better understanding of the neural mechanisms of the analgesic placebo response.

References

Atweh, S. F., and M. J. Kuhar. 1977. "Autoradiographic Ocalization of Opiate Receptors in the Rat Brain. II. The Brain Stem." *Brain Res.,* 129:1–12.

Basbaum, A. I., and H. L. Fields. 1984. "Endogenous Pain Control Systems: Brainstem Spinal Pathways and Endorphin Circuitry." *Annual Rev. Neurosci.,* 7:309–338.

Baskin, D. S., W. R. Mehler, Y. Hosobuchi, D. E. Richardson, and M. A. Flitter. 1986. "Autopsy Analysis of the Safety, Efficacy, and Cartography of Electrical Stimulus of the Central Gray in Humans." *Brain Res.,* 371:231–236.

Beecher, H. K. 1956. "Evidence for Increased Effectiveness of Placebos With Increased Stress." *Am. J. Physiol.,* 187:163–169.

Boivie, J., and B. A. Meyerson. 1982. "A Correlative Anatomical and Clinical Study of Pain Suppression by Deep Brain Stimulation." *Pain,* 13:113–126.

Casey, K. L., S. Minoshima, K. L. Berger, R. A. Koeppe, T. J. Morrow, and K. A. Frey. 1994. "Positron Emission Tomographic Analysis of Cerebral Structures Activated Specifically by Repetitive Noxious Heat Stimuli." *J. Neurophys.,* 71(2):802–807.

Delfs, J. M., H. Kong, A. Mestek, Y. Chen, L. Yu, T. Reisine, and M. F. Chesselet. 1994. "Expression of Mu Ppioid Receptor mRNA in Rat Brain: An *in situ* Hybridization Study at the Single Cell Level." *Journ. Comp. Neurol.,* 345:46–48.

Emson, P. C., R. Corder, S. J. Ratter, S. Tomlin, P. J. Lowry, L. H. Ress, A. Arregui, and M. N. Rosser. 1984. "Regional Distribution of Pro-opiomelanocortin-derived Peptides in the Human Brain." *Neuroendocrinology,* 38(1):45–50.

Evans, F. J. 1985. "Expectancy, Therapeutic Instructions, and the Placebo Response." In L. White, B. Tursky, and G. Schwartz, eds., *Placebo: Theory, Research, and Mechanisms.* New York: Guilford Press, p. 215–228.

Fanselow, M. S. 1984. "Shock-induced Analgesia on the Formalin Test: Effects of Shock Severity, Naloxone, Hypophysectomy, and Associative Variables." *Behav. Neurosci.,* 98(1):79–95.

———. 1991. "The Midbrain Periacqueductal Gray as a Coordinator of

Action in Response to Fear and Anxiety." In A. Depaulis and R. Bandler, eds., *The Midbrain Periacqueductal Gray Matter*. New York: Plenum Press, p. 151–173.

Fedele, L., M. Marchinin, B. Acaia, U. Garagiola, and M. Tiengo. 1989. "Dynamics and Significance of Placebo Response in Primary Dysmenorrhea." *Pain*, 36:43–47.

Fields, H. L., M. M. Heinricher, and P. Mason. 1991. "Neurotransmitters in Nociceptive Modulatory Circuits." *Ann. Rev. Neurosci.*, 14:219–245.

Gelfand, S., L. P. Ullmann, and L. I. Krasner. 1963. "The Placebo Response: An Experimental Approach." *J. Nerv. Mental Diseases*, 136:379–387.

Gracely, R. H., R. Dubner, P. J. Wolskee, and W. R. Deeter. 1983. "Placebo and Naloxone Can Alter Post-surgical Pain by Separate Mechanisms." *Nature*, 306(17):264–265.

Grevert, P., L. H. Albert, and A. Goldstein. 1983a. "Partial Antagonism of Placebo Analgesia by Naloxone." *Pain*, 16:129–143.

Grevert, P., L. H. Albert, C. E. Inturrisi, and A. Goldstein. 1983b. "Effects of Eight-hour Naloxone Infusions on Human Subjects." *Biolog. Psych.*, 18(12):1375–1392.

Grevert, P., and A. Goldstein. 1978. "Endorphins: Naloxone Fails to Alter Experimental Pain or Mood in Humans." *Science*, 199:1093–1095.

———. 1985. "Placebo Analgesia, Naloxone, and the Role of Endogenous Opioids." In L. White, B. Tursky, and G. E. Schwartz, eds., *Placebo: Theory, Research, and Mechanisms*. New York: Guilford Press, p. 332–350.

Helmstetter, F. J., and S. A. Tershner. 1994. "Lesions of the Periacqueductal Gray and Rostral Ventromedial Medulla Disrupt Antinociceptive But Not Cardiovascular Aversive Conditional Responses." *J. Neurosci.*, 14(11):7099–7108.

Kim, J. J., R. A. Rison, and M. S. Fanselow. 1993. "Effects of Amygdala, Hippocampus, and Periaqueductal Gray Lesions on Short- and Long-term Contextual Fear." *Behav. Neurosci.*, 107(6):1093–1098.

Kinscheck, I. B., L. R. Watkins, and D. J. Mayer. 1984. "Fear Is Not Critical to Classically Conditioned Analgesia: The Effects of Periaqueductal Gray Lesions and Administration of Chlorodiazepoxide." *Brain Res.*, 298(1):33–44.

Laska, E., and A. Sunshine. 1973. "Anticipation of Analgesia: A Placebo Effect." *Headache*, 13:1–11.

Lea, S. E., L. Sutton, R. E. Grahn, L. R. Watkins, and S. F. Maier. 1994. "Supersensitivity to Morphine Analgesia Induced by Inescapable Tailshock: Timecourse of Effect." *Abstr. Soc. Neurosci.*, 20(2):964.

Levine, J. D., and N. C. Gordon. 1984. "Influence of the Method of Drug Administration on Analgesic Response." *Nature*, 312(5996):755–756.

Levine, J. D., N. C. Gordon, J. C. Bornstein, and H. L. Fields. 1979. "Role of

Pain in Placebo Analgesia." *Proc. Natl. Acad. Sci. USA*, 76(7):3528–3531.

Levine, J. D., N. C. Gordon, and H. L. Fields. 1978b. "The Mechanism of Placebo Analgesia." *The Lancet*, Sept. 23:654–657.

Levine, J. D., N. C. Gordon, R. T. Jones, and H. L. Fields. 1978a. "The Narcotic Agent Naloxone Enhances Clinical Pain." *Nature*, 272 (5656):826–827.

Levine, J. D., N. C. Gordon, R. Smith, and H. L. Fields. 1981. "Analgesic Responses to Morphine and Placebo in Individuals with Postoperative Pain." *Pain*, 10:379–389.

Liberman, R. 1964. "An Experimental Study of the Placebo Response Under Three Different Situations of Pain." *J. Psychiat. Res.*, 2:233–246.

Lipman, J. J., B. E. Miller, K. S. Mays, M. N. Miller, W. C. North, and W. L. Byrne. 1990. "Peak B Endorphin Concentration in Cerebrospinal Fluid: Reduced in Chronic Pain Patients and Increased During the Placebo Response." *Psychopharmacology*, 102(1):112–116.

Max, M. B., R. K. Portenoy, and E. M. Laska. 1991. *Advances in Pain Research and Therapy, Vol. 18: The Design of Analgesic Clinical Trials.* New York: Raven Press.

Miller, J. S, K. S. Kelly, J. L. Neisewander, D. F. McCoy, M. T. Bardo. 1990. "Conditioning of Morphine-induced Taste Aversion and Analgesia." *Psychopharmacology*, 1990:472–480.

Pitman, R. K., B. A. van der Kolk, S. P. Orr, and M. S. Greenberg. 1990. "Naloxone-Reversible Analgesic Response to Combat-related Stimuli in Posttraumatic Stress Disorder: A Pilot Study." *Arch. Gen. Psychiatry*, 47(6):541–546.

Pittius, C. W., B. R. Seizinger, A. Pasi, P. Mehraein, and A. Herz. 1984. "Distribution and Characterization of Opioid Peptides Derived From Proenkephalin A in Human and Rat Central Nervous System." *Brain Res.*, 304(1):127–136.

Price, D. D. 1988. *Psychological and Neural Mechanisms of Pain.* New York: Raven Press.

Ross, S., and L. W. Buckalew. 1985. "Placebo Agentry: Assessment of Drug and Placebo Effects." In L. White, B. Tursky, and G. E. Schwartz, eds., *Placebo: Theory, Research, and Mechanisms.* New York: Guilford Press, p. 67–82.

Schull, J., H. Kaplan, and C. P. O'Brien. 1981. "Naloxone Can Alter Experimental Pain and Mood in Humans." *Physiol. Proc.*, 9:245–250.

Voudouris, N. J., C. L. Peck, and G. Coleman. 1990. "The Role of Conditioning and Verbal Expectancy in the Placebo Response." *Pain*, 43:121–128.

Wall, P. D. 1994. "The Placebo and the Placebo Response." In P. D. Wall and R. Melzack, eds., *Textbook of Pain*, 3rd ed. New York: Churchill-Livingston, p. 1297–1308.

Watkins, L. R., and D. J. Mayer. 1982. "Organization of Endogenous Opiate and Nonopiate Pain Control Systems." *Science,* 216:1185–1192.

Watkins, L. R., E. G. Young, I. B. Kinscheck, and D. J. Mayer. 1983. "The Neural Basis of Footshock Analgesia: The Role of Specific Ventral Medullary Nuclei." *Brain Res.,* 276:305–315.

White, L., B. Tursky, and G. E. Schwartz, eds. 1985. *Placebo: Theory, Research, and Mechanisms.* New York: Guilford Press.

Wickramasekera, I. 1985. "A Conditioned Response Model of the Placebo Effect: Predictions from the Model." In L. White, B. Tursky, and G. E. Schwartz, eds., *Placebo: Theory, Research, and Mechanisms.* New York: Guilford Press.

Willer, J. C., H. Dehen, and J. Cambier. 1981. "Stress-induced Analgesia in Humans: Endogenous Opioids and Naloxone-reversible Depression of Pain Reflexes." *Science,* 212:689–690.

Willer, J. C., and M. Ernst. 1986. "Diazepam Reduces Stress-induced Analgesia in Humans." *Brain Res.,* 362:398–402.

Wolkowitz, O. M., and J. R. Tinklenberg. 1985. "Naloxone's Effects on Cognitive Functioning in Drug-free and Diazepam-treated Normal Humans." *Psychopharmacology,* 85(2):221–223.

Yaksh, T. L., N. R. F. Al-Rodhan, and T. X. Jensen. 1988. "Sites of Action of Opiates in Production of Analgesia." *Prog. Brain Res.,* 77:371–394.

Acknowledgments

The authors thank Jon Levine, Mary Heinricher, and Gabriel Fields for their detailed critical review of this manuscript, and Laura Harger for editorial assistance. Supported by NIH grants DA01949 and NS21445.

The Contribution of Desire and Expectation to Placebo Analgesia: Implications for New Research Strategies

6

Donald D. Price
Howard L. Fields

Under conditions wherein patients have a strong need to be relieved of pain and/or they have expectations that pain relief will occur as a result of a treatment, and/or the treatment situation reproduces in some way a previously effective treatment, pain reduction may result from psychological factors. This constitutes the placebo analgesic response. A better understanding of how placebo manipulations, such as saline injections, can reduce pain requires explicit attention to determine which dimensions of pain are most affected by such manipulations and what are the most important psychological factors that contribute to the placebo effect.

In this chapter, a strategy is recommended for future studies of pain reduction produced by placebo manipulations. This strategy should lead to an improvement in both the analysis of the psychological variables likely to constitute mediating factors in placebo analgesia as well as the analysis of dimensions of pain influenced by placebo treatments. On the basis of the available literature, we propose that two general factors mediate placebo analgesia: (1) *a desire or need for relief of pain* and (2) *an expectation that a given procedure or agent will relieve the pain.* In the context of providing support for a two-factor model that includes these dimensions, the following relevant questions are addressed: (1) What environmental or situational factors influence the magnitude of the placebo response? (2) Given these environmental factors, what is the role of classical conditioning in placebo analgesia? (3) How do psychological factors such as anxiety, belief, hope, desire

117

for pain relief, and expectancy relate to these environmental factors and contribute to placebo analgesia? And (4) how could one optimally measure and assess the relative contributions of *desire for relief of pain* and *expectation* in producing effects on the different dimensions of pain?

Environmental and Situational Factors

There are two general lines of evidence that support the idea that placebo analgesic effects are influenced by degree of threat that is present in the context in which placebo treatments are given. The first is based on comparisons of placebo analgesic effects across studies of different types of pain. Both Beecher (1955; 1959) and Jospe (1978) asserted that the magnitudes of analgesic response to an explicit placebo manipulation are, in general, much greater in studies of clinical pain than in studies of experimental pain. Although both authors base this assertion on considerable numbers of studies, a serious limitation in this comparison is that the natural history of the patients'/subjects' pain is rarely taken into account in clinical studies (for further discussion, see Chapter 5). However, among studies utilizing experimental pain, for which assessments of the natural history and/or baseline reliability are more often provided, placebo analgesic effects are larger for those forms of experimental pain that are of longer duration and/or are more stressful (Jospe 1978). These types of experimental pain are more likely to simulate the psychological conditions of most acute clinical pains. Thus, whereas placebo treatment produces large reductions in experimental limb ischemic pain which continuously increases in intensity over several minutes (Grevert et al. 1983; Grevert and Goldstein 1985), placebo has no effect on brief pains produced by five-second heat stimuli (Price et al. 1985; 1988).

The second line of evidence, closely related to the first, is the general relationship between pain intensity and placebo analgesia. Beecher (1955; 1959) found that pain relief from the same dose of morphine decreased as a function of pain intensity, whereas placebo responses increased as a function of pain intensity (Beecher 1955; 1959). Unfortunately, the lack of no-treatment groups in these studies casts some doubt on this finding. Levine et al. (1979) provided evidence that supports a threshold level for placebo analgesia and hence a relationship between pain level and placebo effect. If one assumes that the severity of the pain contributes significantly to the experienced need for pain relief, a direct relationship between placebo effect and pain intensity indirectly indicates that the placebo response increases as a function of this need. Thus, in situations wherein pain itself serves as a strong threat or in emergency situations wherein both severe pain and other threats are experienced, placebo responses should be optimized. It is important to point out that situational factors that influence perceived threat are likely to vary considerably according to the external circumstances of the patient as well as to the specific meanings given to these circumstances by the patient. These factors are likely to contribute to the large variability in mean magnitude of the placebo effect across studies (Jospe 1978; White et al. 1985). Systematic differences in natural history across different types of pain may also have contributed to this variability (see Chapter 5).

The Contribution of Learning

It would be surprising indeed if factors related to learning were not involved in the placebo response. After all, it is common clinical experience that patients learn to expect therapeutic effects from various treatments. A number of psychologists have independently proposed that the placebo response can be at least partly explained on the basis of classical conditioning, thereby providing a formal testable scientific model for the role of learning in the placebo response. Wickramasekera (1985) proposes that active ingredients of agents that reduce pain (morphine, aspirin, and so forth) can serve as unconditioned stimuli (UCS), whereas neutral stimuli associated with the *diminution* of unpleasant symptoms (due to spontaneous remission or delivery of an active drug) or with the *onset* of therapeutic action of an active ingredient for therapeutic effects can serve as conditioned stimuli (CS). CS are those stimuli that can be associated with the therapeutic agent and its efficacy, such as syringes, authoritative-appearing healthcare professionals, elaborate medical equipment, and so on. CSs may also operate to potentiate healing by indicating that the period of suffering is over or that prospects for recovery have increased (Mowrer 1960).

Wickramasekera draws many parallels between characteristics of classically conditioned behavior and aspects of the placebo response to support his explanation. For example, the conditioned response (CR) to placebo manipulations (CS) should have a smaller magnitude than the unconditioned response (UCR) to the active ingredients of the therapeutic agent. The classical conditioning model predicts that therapists who use UCSs or active ingredients will get stronger placebo effects than those who use only CSs or neutral ingredients, because regular UCS-CS association strenthens the CR. Karcyn (1978) has made a similiar explanation based on theoretical grounds. The applicability of the classical conditioning model to the placebo response is indirectly supported by empirical observations that analgesia associated with conditioned fear in rats can be classically conditioned (see Watkins and Mayer 1982; Chapter 5, this volume). On the basis of this finding, Watkins and Mayer reasoned that placebo analgesia might also be subserved by classical conditioning wherein repeated administration of a drug would serve as the UCS. The analgesic response to the drug and to the placebo would serve as the UCR and the CR respectively.

Human studies also clearly show that prior experience with an effective analgesic drug enhances the analgesic effectiveness of a subsequent placebo. To take one of the more salient examples from the literature, Laska and Sunshine (1973) designed a clinical trial in which a second medication, always placebo, followed graded doses of propxyphene HCL (3 dose levels), propoxyphene napsylate (3 doses), or placebo. Thus, there were seven groups of patients with fourteen to twenty patients in each group. Their results showed convincing evidence of a "dose-response relationship" between the dose of the first medication and the analgesic response to the subsequent placebo, though the magnitudes of placebo effects were lower than their corresponding doses of the active drug. Placebo given as a second treatment acted as an effective analgesic when it followed an effective analgesic, whereas placebo following a placebo continued to have the same slight analgesic effect as the first placebo had. One can easily interpret their results as supportive of learning, even classical conditioning (see Chapter 5). However, the authors themselves conclude that the time course of the pain plus the *anticipation* of relief based on past experience probably combine in some complex and highly individualized subtle way to produce their pattern of results.

There have been several challenges to explaining placebo effects on the basis of classical (Pavlovian) conditioning. In particular, Kirsch (1990) has pointed out that various studies of placebo effects have failed several criteria that are used to decide whether a phenomenon can be attributed to classical conditioning: (1) conditioning trials with tranquilizers weaken rather than produce the predicted strengthened placebo effect; (2) contrary to the criterion that the magnitude of placebo effect should be directly related to the strength of the active tranquilizer, it is *inversely related;* (3) the placebo effects are often not specific to the pharmacological properties of the active drug (for example, alcohol, caffeine) but depend heavily on context and suggestion; (4) placebos often fail the extinction test as in the case of placebo treatment for panic disorder; (5) placebo effects sometimes can be stronger (not weaker) than the effects of an active drug. On the other hand, except for the demonstration of extinction, all of of the criteria for classical conditioning are fulfilled by the Laska and Sunshine study just discussed. As well, Fedele et al. (1989) demonstrated a loss of analgesic effectiveness of placebo with repeated administration (that is, extinction). The exceptions cited by Kirsch may be unique to certain kinds of studies in which psychologically therapeutic effects are measured (for example, reductions in panic or anxiety) or to instances wherein a drug induces arousal or sedation (that is, caffeine or alcohol) but in which the specific effects observed, such as increased motor performance, could be attributed largely to contextual factors and suggestion. These considerations may have less application to placebo analgesia, at least to its sensory-discriminative dimension.

The Contribution of Cognitive Factors

The study of cognitive factors has the potential for increasing understanding of how learning influences the placebo effect and how factors not directly related to classical conditioning influence placebo responses. First of all, CSs and CRs may well have concomitant cognitive dimensions. For example, CSs occurring during the visit to the doctor and during the prescription and ingestion of medication, such as pills and syringes, become associated with active pharmacological agents, UCSs, as well as with the reduction in pain (UCR). They can indicate that the period of pain, uncertainty, fear, and depression is over and/or that relief and healing are imminent.

While the consideration of cognitive factors extends and supports the role of learning and even classical conditioning in placebo analgesia, cognitive factors also help to resolve some of the limitations and inconsistencies of classical conditioning as an explanation for placebo analgesia. Although there is ample evidence that prior exposure to an effective treatment enhances placebo effects, it is not clear that such prior exposure is a necessary condition for a placebo response. Because of the important roles that meanings, attributions, imagery, and information have in mediating beliefs, desires, and expectations, it is plausible that the placebo response is more directly controlled by these cognitive factors than by the immediate and direct association of a specific treatment with pain reduction as required for classical conditioning (i.e., "conditioned and unconditioned stimuli").

Indeed, consideration of the nature of suggestions inherent in placebo manipulations strongly indicate that cognitive factors operate to influence and even determine the nature and magnitude of the placebo response. The "suggestion" provided in the case of placebo analgesia has a meaning that is more specific than that of suggestion in general and can be distinguished from other forms of suggestion, such as that provided during hypnotic analgesia. The suggestion in placebo analgesia is to the effect that pain relief is being provided from an outside authoritative source (for instance, pain medicine prescribed by a knowledgeable professional). Within the placebo literature, there exists evidence that greater placebo effects are achieved by more believable and more technically convincing agents. Thus, it is claimed that placebo injections are more effective than placebo pills and that placebo morphine is more effective than placebo aspirin (Traut and Passarelli 1957). Implicit in the overall suggestion inherent to a placebo analgesic manipulation is the idea that in the absence of this outside authoritative agent, there would indeed be unrelieved pain. The nature of hypnotic suggestions for analgesia differs from that of placebo in that hypnotic suggestions for analgesia refer to a more innate and self-directed capacity to experience pain differently, often to the effect that one can experience sensations differently, including the possibility that there is no pain to be experienced (Barber and Adrian 1982). What may be developed in the case of placebo analgesia, then, is a different class of expectation, that is, that an acceptable therapeutic agent will provide significant relief of pain. All of these types of suggestion are learned, regardless of whether or not they reflect the intentions of the person who administers them.

The Role of Expectation

This possible role of *expectation* in placebo responses is supported both by new alternative models of learning (Reiss 1980) and by some evidence that expectation plays a critical role in the placebo response. Recognizing that classical conditioning itself may reflect a cognitive process, Reiss argues, "What is learned in Pavlovian conditioning is an expectation regarding the occurrence or nonoccurrence of a UCS onset or a change in UCS magnitude or duration." However, although classical conditioning is one way in which to change one's expectation, other types of learning can contribute. For example, expectation can reflect knowledge about the therapeutic agent, the circumstances under which it is administered, and the condition which is to be treated. Classical conditioning could result in increased knowledge about the efficacy of the therapeutic agent by producing a memory of past effects. On the other hand, one could also read a book about the agent's therapeutic efficacy. In either case, increased information indicating an agent's effectiveness could increase one's expectation of relief.

What all of this implies for placebo analgesia is that *expectation* for relief may cause a placebo response without prior exposure to a therapeutic agent, though such exposure certainly will increase expectation (for example, Laska and Sunshine 1973). This possibility is supported by several studies that indirectly show that expectation exerts a considerable influence in the production of placebo effects. Lasagna et al. (1958) analyzed postoperative patients who responded to placebos and to analgesic drugs. They concluded that a positive placebo response indicates a psychological set wherein pain relief is anticipated. Unfortunately, neither the early studies of placebo analgesia by Beecher's group nor most of the recent studies of placebo analgesia have directly assessed the role of expectation. Although the study of Nash and Zimring (1969) focused on effects of placebo on short-term memory and not pain, they specifically studied the role of expectation in one hundred patients. They compared effects of two drugs versus placebo and found that the two drugs had no effect that differentiated them from placebo. However, there was a strong correlation between the measured expectation and the placebo effect. Importantly, though both correlations were statistically reliable, the correlation was stronger for subjectively experienced change in performance of memory tests ($R = 0.36$) than for objective tests of performance ($R = 0.23$).

Despite the commonly asserted claim that expectation constitutes a critical factor in placebo effects, its role has not been consistently demonstrated in experiments explicitly designed to assess its relative contribution, particularly in analgesic studies. Furthermore, the effects of expectation on placebo analgesia have yet to be convincingly distinguished from those of conditioning. These uncertainties are evident in the work of Voudouris et al (1990), who compared effects of *conditioning* (exposure to a "pain-reducing treatment") and explicit *expectation* (verbal suggestions for pain reduction) manipulations within the same experiment on placebo analgesia. There were four groups in the study: Group 1 received a combined *expectancy* and *conditioning* manipulation; Group 2 received *expectancy* treatment alone; Group 3 received *conditioning* alone; Group 4, a control group, received neither treatment. All subject's Visual Analog Scale (VAS) ratings of pain were compared with and without a placebo cream, using iontophoretic pain stimulation. Their results showed an enhanced placebo effect from *conditioning* but not *expectancy* and no interaction between the two different types of manipulations. The authors suggest that conditioning may be a more powerful factor than verbal expectancy in inducing a placebo response.

Although this study was the first attempt to assess the differential role of conditioning and expectancy in evoking placebo analgesia, there are several problems with this study that are specifically related to the expectancy manipulation and its assessment. In the first place, the expectancy manipulation itself is questionable because it consisted of simply providing different consent forms for the expectancy groups and the conditioning-alone group, one form stating that group members would receive a powerful analgesic and the other form stating that they were in a control group. Whether this approach was actually effective among the university students who participated, given their possible level of knowledge of psychology experiments, is open to question. Secondly, their expectancy manipulation check was simplistic, consisting of an analysis of responses to only a single question (embedded in a series of other irrelevant questions) asking "whether they expected this cream to be effective." Finally, they asked this question only once, *prior* to the conditioning manipulation. Thus, the effect of conditioning on expectancy was never assessed. As is appropriate given these problems, the authors indicate that their results by no means exclude a role of expectation in evoking placebo responses. Rather, they suggest that expectations may be more strongly shaped by previous experience (such as that provided by conditioning) than by verbal persuasion. The authors admit that it would have been more revealing to have actually directly assessed the expectation levels of subjects who received only conditioning rather than simply to have assumed expectation was successfully increased only by their expectancy manipulation. Direct measures of expectation by means of continuous scales or questionnaires with multiple questions about expectation clearly need to be incorporated into studies of placebo effects. These measures may account for more of the variance in placebo effects than the manipulations intended to produce changes in expectation.

The Role of Desire for Relief, or Motivation

Although expectation may be a salient factor that influences the magnitude of the placebo response, it does not appear to operate alone. Placebo effects are commonly observed in circumstances wherein it is likely that subjects not only expect therapeutic effects but also strongly want these effects to occur. Although desire for relief, or motivation, which is not quite the same thing, has been directly or indirectly implicated in the placebo response, less explicit recognition has been given to this factor than to that of expectation. In one exceptional study of placebo manipulations suggesting possible sedative or stimulant effects, Jensen and Karoly (1991) assessed the separate contributions of *motivation* and *expectancy* to placebo responses. They manipulated both of these factors by separate instructions and then later checked (by subject self-ratings) to determine whether either factor or both factors had been influenced. Thus, the study was a 2 × 2 factorial design which contained four groups (high motivation-high expectancy, and so on). They found that motivation accounted for a significant amount of variance in the placebo responses that included both perceived sedation or stimulant effect but obtained equivocal results from expectation. Nevertheless, they maintained that both factors are likely to contribute to placebo responses.

The Possible Implicit Nature of Desire and Expectation

Although there exists some experimental support for the roles of motivation and expectation in the placebo response, there remains uncertainty as to whether patients/subjects are fully aware of these factors or whether they are *implicit* and in the background of one's experience. Thus, both desire for relief and expectation may occur implicitly in the form of imagery. Kojo (1988) suggests that imagery operates in placebo phenomena in much the same way that thermal imagery operates to increase blood flow and skin temperature. Imaging one's hand as warm for several seconds or minutes can result in actual increases in blood flow and skin temperature. Kojo suggests that the content of treatment-induced imagery *and* the associated physiological changes constitute the placebo effect. Strongly wanting and expecting the desired therapeutic effects may lead to images related to perception of the therapeutic effects themselves. These images may be the "figures" of experience, whereas the desire and expectations that support them remain as "ground." The presence of these experiential factors may be discerned by methods that uncover what is implicit in experience (Merleau-Ponty 1962). Phenomenological approaches that utilize methods of passive observation and experiential self-reporting can be used to identify common elements of human experiences (Price and Barrell 1980). Therefore, it may be worthwhile to study the presence or absence of the factors of *desire for relief* and *expectation* retrospectively or prospectively and to obtain multiple measures of these factors in future placebo experiments. Furthermore, since these two cognitive factors are likely to interact in combination, it is essential to measure both.

The potential implicit nature of desire and expectation also relates to the question of whether these experiential factors or classical conditioning (independent of expectation) operate to produce placebo effects. After all, it is possible that placebo effects occur in people without conscious awareness of the critical factors that produce them. If experiments designed to assess simultaneously the roles of conditioning, of desire for relief, and of expectation fail to show effects of the latter two factors, then the hypothesis that classical conditioning independent of expectation and desire produces placebo effects would be supported. However, a fair test of both possibilities requires much more thorough attempts to assess the contribution of expectation and desire than has been carried out to date.

Analysis of Factors That Help to Explain the Placebo Effect

Nearly all studies that have sought to explain the psychological basis of the placebo effect have focused on a single factor such as anxiety, expectancy, hope, or faith in the treatment. On the basis of the studies and considerations previously elaborated, we propose that three factors need to be explicitly tested for their possible contribution to placebo analgesia. These include (1) a classical conditioning effect that occurs without the subject's conscious awareness of the CS-UCS association; (2) a desire for a given treatment or agent to significantly relieve pain; and, (3) the level of expectation that pain will be significantly relieved by such treatment or agent. Although we think that classical conditioning is a major determinant of the magnitude of the placebo effect, we propose that a combination of desire and expectation can be of equal if not greater importance.

Repeated treatments that are efficacious in reducing pain lead to increased expectations for relief. However, while repetition of the treatments and hence conditioning may be sufficient for such an effect, it may not be necessary. Cognitive influences that have a direct, immediate, and unique impact on one's expectation for relief can occur without prior exposure to the treatment under question. Thus, the model also accounts for the several studies that suggest that *expectation* is a salient determinant of placebo analgesia (Laska and Sunshine 1973; White et al. 1985).

Desire for a specific treatment or agent to produce relief of pain also accounts for several observations. It accounts for the increase in placebo response with the severity of clinical pain. It also accounts for the greater placebo response for clinical pain versus experimental pain and for the observation that placebo responses in experimental pain increase as a function of its duration and severity. In other words, the greater and more open-ended is the threat related to the pain, the greater the need for relief and the greater the placebo response.

The combination of both factors may account for the association between the placebo response and anxiety. Anxiety represents a combination of desire to avoid negative consequences coupled with an uncertain expectation of avoiding those consequences (Price and Barrell 1980; Price et al. 1985). These two dimensions comprise the anxiety that is associated with acute clinical pain. To the extent that patients increase their expectation that a given treatment or agent will reduce their pain, their anxiety decreases when they receive the treatment. This reduction in anxiety would be expected to reduce the unpleasantness associated with pain (Price 1988).

Finally, the two factors of desire and expectation extend the theoretical position of Plotkin (1985) that "faith" or "hope" constitutes much of the basis for the placebo response. Concepts of "faith" or "hope" implicitly contain the dimensions of need or desire and expectation, dimensions which though interrelated are separate (Price et al. 1985). To have hope is to have an expectation whose level is greater than that of "impossibility." However, expectation lacks emotional feeling if it is not coupled with the desire for a particular outcome and is not sufficient for hope. If these two factors contribute, one might expect that the placebo response is accompanied by emotions or changes in emotions, since desire and expectation are essential elements for many basic human emotions (Price and Barrell 1984; Price et al. 1985; Price 1988).

Implications of the Desire/Expectation Model for Assessment of Placebo Analgesia in Clinical and Experimental Contexts

So far, the approach in demonstrating effects of conditioning or expectation on placebo analgesia has been to provide explicit instructions or experimental manipulations that one can assume increase a patient's expectation that a treatment will relieve pain. However, in all such studies, the manipulations themselves constitute the independent variables of the experiment. Measures of expectation or motivation have been used to determine whether the manipulations were effective and not as independent variables themselves. The Nash and Zimring study (1969), which focused on memory and not pain, showed significant correlations between placebo effects and expectation ratings (see earlier). No one has yet reported using direct rating or questionnaire response measures of either desire or expectation as independent variables in a study of placebo analgesia. However, if these two factors are salient in mediating placebo analgesia, then it should be possible to measure them and assign them as independent variables in placebo studies. Are there methods available for directly measuring patients'/subjects' strength of desire to be relieved of pain and their expectation that a given therapy or agent will bring significant relief?

The capacity to use direct scaling techniques to measure desire and expectation as independent variables in an experiment is demonstrated in studies of human emotions (Price and Barrell 1984; Price et al. 1985). Psychophysical methods were used to develop scales for both desirability of an outcome and expectation about its occurrence. Importantly, visual analog scales and line production scaling procedures first demonstrated that ratio scales could be developed for the factors of *expectation* and *desire for a specific outcome* (Price and Barrell 1984). These factors were then shown to have lawful interactions in their influence on the magnitudes of both positive and negative emotional feelings. The magnitude of positive and negative feeling intensity was shown to be a multiplicative function of *both* desire for an outcome and its perceived likelihood (expectation) of occurrence. The nature of this multiplicative interaction also was influenced by whether the goal was that of avoiding negative consequences (an *avoidance* goal) or obtaining pleasurable or satisfying consequences (an *approach* goal).

As can be discerned from Figure 6.1, emotional feeling intensity was a positively accelerating function of expectation in the case of *avoidance* goals (Feeling intensity = Desire $\times$ Expectation^2), whereas emotional feeling intensity was a negatively accelerating function of expectation in the case of *approach* goals (Feeling intensity = Desire $\times$ Expectation$^{.5}$). These factors and their interrelationships were further used to characterize human emotions such as depression, anxiety, excitement, and satisfaction. For example, anxiety was associated with *avoidance* goals and and expectation levels within the middle of the expectation range (Figure 6.1). If such precise interactions between desire and expectation can be demonstrated in the case of human emotions, it should be possible to demonstrate their interactions and influence in other phenomena such as the effects of placebo. This possibility seems reasonable, given the claimed associations between human emotions and placebo effects, for example between anxiety reduction and placebo effect (Evans 1985).

Thus, studies of placebo effects could utilize manipulations that are intended separately to influence either desire for a therapeutic effect or expectation, and such studies could have two sets of independent variables: one set would be the manipulations intended to alter the critical variables, and the other set would be ratings of desire and expectation. The advantage of using visual analogue scale ratings of desire and expectation is that they constitute continuous ratio scale measures and could be applied in both clinical and experimental settings. Moreover, if the manipulation was that of conditioning, then the experiment could be designed to distinguish whether the conditioning manipulation itself or the experiential factors best accounted for the variance in placebo effects.

Using this approach, one could, for example, determine whether an additive or multiplicative model of the desire/expectation interaction accounts for more of the variance in placebo response. The question of whether an additive or multiplicative model of these factors best accounts for the variance in placebo effects is both testable and heuristic. For example, it may be that high levels of expectation are sufficient to

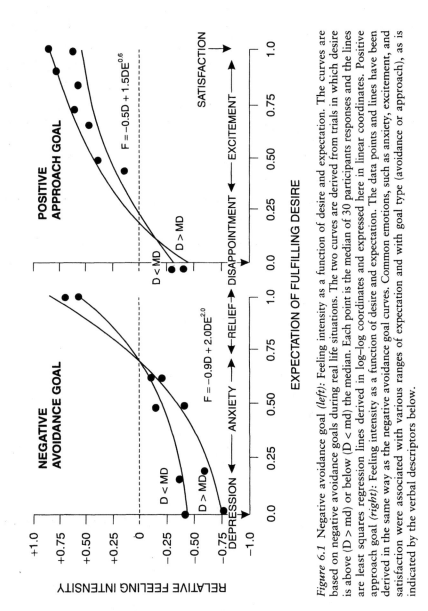

Figure 6.1 Negative avoidance goal *(left)*: Feeling intensity as a function of desire and expectation. The curves are based on negative avoidance goals during real life situations. The two curves are derived from trials in which desire is above (D > md) or below (D < md) the median. Each point is the median of 30 participants responses and the lines are least squares regression lines derived in log–log coordinates and expressed here in linear coordinates. Positive approach goal *(right)*: Feeling intensity as a function of desire and expectation. The data points and lines have been derived in the same way as the negative avoidance goal curves. Common emotions, such as anxiety, excitement, and satisfaction were associated with various ranges of expectation and with goal type (avoidance or approach), as is indicated by the verbal descriptors below.

induce placebo side effects even when these side effects are neither desirable nor undesirable. Such a result would be consistent with the additive model of Desire and Expectation. On the other hand, if critical levels of both desire and expectation are necessary for placebo effects and if these factors interact to an extent that is much greater than that predicted by the sum of their values, then a multiplicative model could apply. It would be interesting indeed if a Desire × Expectation model shown to be applicable to human emotions also applied to placebo effects. The nature of this interactive effect of desire and expectation on placebo responses might also differ according to whether the subject's desired therapeutic effect represents an *avoidance* or *approach* goal, similiar to human emotions (Figure 6.1). Thus, placebo effects of analgesia, associated with the desire to reduce and hence avoid pain, may require higher levels of expectation than that required for placebo effects of euphoria, assuming that euphoria represents an approach goal.

Analysis of Effects of These Factors on Multiple Dimensions of Pain

Just as there are multiple psychological dimensions or factors that contribute to placebo responses, the placebo responses themselves are likely to comprise multiple dimensions. Pain has both a sensory-discriminative and an affective-motivational dimension. The strategy previously discussed for characterizing the critical psychological factors that mediate placebo analgesia could be interfaced with one which assesses how these factors influence the different dimensions of pain.

The potential strength of this strategy requires that accurate, sensitive, and valid methods of pain measurement be used. This requirement may be accomplished by using pain measurement methods that fulfill criteria for ideal pain measurement (Gracely and Dubner 1981; Price 1988). Direct magnitude scaling of sensory and affective dimensions of pain would seem essential, especially if placebo effects differentially influence the two dimensions of pain. Turskey (1985) has recommended the use of more sophisticated scaling methods and has pointed out the deficiencies of category and other assessment methods as they relate to the assessment of placebo effects.

Studies That Separately Measure Pain Sensation and Pain Affect

Under some circumstances, placebo effects in pain patients may involve only a reduction in anxiety and therefore a selective reduction in the affective dimension of pain. Such a selective antianxiety effect could occur if the patient were led to expect that the therapeutic agent would make the pain less threatening, bothersome, or distressing but not necessarily less intense (for example, "I am going to give you something to make it easier to tolerate the pain"). The patient's expectation that the agent will have such an effect might in itself reduce anxiety both before and after a painful procedure, thereby reducing both the anxiety of anticipating pain and the unpleasantness of the pain. Thus far, only one study has shown a selective effect of a placebo on the affective dimension of pain. Gracely (1979) found that saline placebo reduced affective but not sensory ratings of experimental pain, and that this effect was greater toward the low end of the nociceptive stimulus range. This pattern of effect is similiar to that produced by diazepam, an anxiety-reducing agent (Gracely et al. 1976) and by cognitive manipulations that are likely to reduce anxiety (Price and Barrell 1980).

It is very unlikely that all placebo manipulations selectively influence the affective dimension of pain by reducing anxiety. In fact, such a possibility is inconsistent with the observation that placebo effects are larger for severe pain as compared with mild pain, a pattern at variance with Gracely et al.'s (1976) finding that an antianxiety agent reduced the unpleasantness of mild but not more intense pain. It is also inconsistent with other studies showing placebo effects on sensory intensive aspects of pain (Grevert and Goldstein 1985; Levine et al. 1978) and the reversal of these effects by naloxone. The possibility must be considered that there are multiple placebo analgesic effects. Clearly, different desires and expectations could be induced in patients/subjects by the way in which placebo suggestions are framed, and even the same placebo instructions could lead some people to expect reductions in unpleasantness and others to expect reductions in both pain sensation intensity and unpleasantness. These possibilities are indirectly supported by studies of hypnotic analgesia wherein different subjects show vastly different proportions of reductions in pain-affect and pain-sensation intensity (Price and Barber 1987; Kiernan et al. 1994). The hypothesis that, under some circumstances, placebos reduce pain unpleasantness by reducing anxiety needs to be tested directly by methods that directly assess anxiety as well as sensory and affective dimensions of pain.

Implications for Future Analyses of Placebo Analgesia

Knowledge about the psychological and neural mechanisms by which placebo treatments reduce pain has far-reaching implications for treatment of medical conditions, including pain. For example, suppose it is true that a specific kind of placebo reduces pain intensity and not just the unpleasantness or even one's bias in rating pain. The reduction of pain intensity by a placebo administration implies that the physiological consequences of pain, such as reduced immune response and prolongation of healing, also would be ameliorated (Liebeskind 1991). In this way, placebo treatments have the potential for influencing physiological and pathophysiological processes of the body, including those related to cancer. As another example, suppose the experiential factors that are neccessary and sufficient for the placebo effect become established and well-characterized. Knowledge of these factors could then be more directly and optimally utilized by both patients and healthcare providers. The concept of "placebo manipulations" would shift in emphasis from reliance on outside authority to the patients' active participation in developing optimal psychological conditions for therapeutic effects.

References

Barber, J., and C. Adrian. 1982. *Psychological Approaches to the Management of Pain*. New York: Brunner/Mazel.

Beecher, H. K. 1955. "The Powerful Placebo." *J. Amer. Med. Ass.,* 159:1602–1606.

————. 1959. *Measurement of Subjective Responses: Quantitative Effects of Drugs*. New York: Oxford University Press.

Bootzin, R. R. 1985. "The Role of Expectancy in Behavior Change." In L.

White, B. Tursky, and G. E. Schwartz, eds., *Placebo: Theory, Research, and Mechanisms.* New York: Guilford Press.

Evans, F. J. 1985. "Expectancy, Therapeutic Instructions, and the Placebo Response." In L. White, B. Tursky, and G. E. Schwartz, eds., *Placebo: Theory, Research, and Mechanisms.* New York: Guilford Press.

Fedele, L., M. Marchinin, B. Acaia, U. Garagiola, and M. Tiengo. 1989. "Dynamics and Significance of Placebo Response in Primary Dysmenor-rhea." *Pain,* 36:43–47.

Fields, H. L., and A. I. Basbaum. 1994. "Endogenous Pain Control Mecha-nisms." In P. D. Wall and R. Melzack, eds., *Textbook of Pain,* 3rd ed., Edinburgh: Churchill Livingston.

Goldstein, A., and E. R. Hilgard. 1975. "Lack of Influence of the Morphine Antagonist Naloxone on Hypnotic Analgesia." *Proceeding of the Na-tional Academy of Science,* 72:2041–2043.

Gracely, R. H. 1979. "Psychophysical Assessment of Human Pain." In J. J. Bonica, J. C. Liebeskind, and D. G. Albe-Fessard, eds. *Advances in Pain Research and Therapy,* Vol. 3. New York: Raven Press.

Gracely, R. H., and R. Dubner. 1981. "Pain Assessment in Humans—A Reply to Hall." *Pain,* 11:109–120.

Gracely, R. H., P. McGrath, and R. Dubner. 1976. "Validity and Sensitivity of Ratio Scales of Sensory and Affective Verbal Pain Descriptors: Manipu-lation of Affect by Diazepam." *Pain,* 2:19–29.

Grevert, P., L. H. Albert, and A. Goldstein. 1983. "Partial Analgesia by Naloxone." *Pain,* 16:129–143.

Grevert, P., and A. Goldstein. 1985. "Placebo Analgesia, Naloxone, and the Role of Endogenous Opioids." In L. White, B. Tursky, and G. E. Schwartz, eds., *Placebo: Theory, Research, and Mechanisms.* New York: Guilford Press.

Hilgard, E. R., and J. R. Hilgard. 1983. *Hypnosis in the Relief of Pain.* Los Altos, Calif.: William Kaufmann, p. 294.

Jensen, M. P., and P. Karoly. 1991. "Motivation and Expectancy Factors in Symptom Perception: A Laboratory Study of the Placebo Effect." *Psy-chosom. Med.,* 53:144–152.

Jospe, M. 1978. *The Placebo Effect in Healing.* Lexington, Mass.: Lexington Books.

Karcyn, A. D. 1978. "Mechanism of Placebo Analgesia." *Lancet,* 2:1304–1305.

Kiernan, B. D., J. R. Dane, L. H. Phillips, and D. D. Price. 1994. "Hypnotic Analgesia Reduces R-III Nociceptive Reflex: Further Evidence Concerning the Multifactorial Nature of Hypnotic Analgesia." *Pain* (In Press).

Kirsch, I. 1990. *Changing Expectations: A Key to Effective Psychotherapy.* Pacific Grove, Calif.: Brooks/Cole.

Kojo, I. 1988. "The Mechanism of Psychophysiological Effects of Placebo." *Medical Hypotheses,* 27:261–264.

Lasagna, L., V. G. Laties, and J. L. Dohan. 1958. "Further Studies on the 'Pharmacology' of a Placebo Administration." *J. Clin. Invest.*, 37:533–537.

Laska, E., and A. Sunshine. 1973. "Anticipation of Analgesia a Placebo Effect." *Headache*, 13:1–11.

Levine, J. D., N. C. Gordon, and H. L. Fields. 1978. "The Mechanism of Placebo Analgesia." *Lancet*, 2:654–657.

Levine, J. D., N. C. Gordon, J. C. Bornstein, and H. L. Fields. 1979. "Role of Pain in Placebo Analgesia." *PNAS*, 76:3528–3531.

Liebeskind, J. C. 1991. "Pain Can Kill." *Pain*, 44:3–4.

Melzack, R., and K. L. Casey. 1968. "Sensory, Motivational, and Central Control of Determinants of Pain." In Kenshalo, ed., *The Skin Sense*. Springfield, Ill.: Charles C. Thomas, p. 423–439.

Merleau-Ponty, M. 1962. *The Phenomenology of Perception*. New York: The Humanities Press.

Mowrer, O. H. 1960. *Learning Theory and Behavior*. New York: Wiley.

Nash, N. N., and F. M. Zimring. 1969. "Prediction of Reaction to Placebo." *J. of Abnormal Psychology*, 74:569–573.

Plotkin, W. B. 1985. "A Psychological Approach to Placebo: The Role of Faith in Therapy and Treatment." In L. White, B. Tursky, and G. E. Schwartz, eds., *Placebo: Theory, Research, and Mechanisms*. New York: Guilford Press.

Price, D. D. 1988. *Psychological and Neural Mechanisms of Pain*. New York: Raven Press.

Price, D. D., and J. Barber. 1987. "An Analysis of Factors That Contribute to the Efficacy of Hypnotic Analgesia." *J. Abn. Psychol*, 96:46–51.

Price, D. D., and J. J. Barrell. 1980. "An Experiential Approach with Quantitative Methods: A Research Paradigm." *J. Humanistic Psychology*, 20:75–95.

———. 1984. "Some General Laws of Human Emotion: Interrelationships Between Intensities of Desire, Expectation, and Emotional Feeling." *J. Personality*, 52(4):389–409.

Price, D. D., J. E. Barrell, and J. J. Barrell. 1985. "A Quantitative-experiential Analysis of Human Emotions." *Motivation and Emotions*, 9:19–38.

Price, D. D., J. J. Barrell, and R. H. Gracely. 1980. "A Psychophysical Analysis of Experiential Factors That Selectively Influence the Affective Dimension of Pain." *Pain*, 8:137–179.

Reiss, S. 1980. "Pavlovian Conditioning and Human Fear: An Expectancy Model." *Behavior Therapy*, 11:380–396.

Schacter, S., and J. Singer. 1962. "Cognitive, Social, and Physiological Determinants of the Emotional State." *Psychol. Rev.*, 36:379–399.

Traut, E. F., and E. W. Passarelli. 1957. "Placebos in the Treatment of

Rheumatoid Arthritis and Other Rheumatic Conditions." *Annals of the Rheumatic Diseases,* 16:18–22.

Turskey, B. 1985. "The 55% Analgesic Effect: Real or Artifact?" In L. White, B. Tursky, and G. E. Schwartz, eds., *Placebo: Theory, Research, and Mechanisms.* New York: Guilford Press.

Voudouris, N. J., C. L. Peck, and G. Coleman. 1990. "The Role of Conditioning and Expectancy in the Placebo Response." *Pain,* 43:121–128.

Watkins, L. R., and D. J. Mayer. 1982. "Organization of Endogenous Opiate and Nonopiate Pain Control Systems." *Science,* 216:1185–1192.

White, L., B. Tursky, and G. E. Schwartz, eds. 1985. *Placebo: Theory, Research, and Mechanisms.* New York: Guilford Press.

Wickramasekera, I. 1985. "A Conditioned Response Model of the Placebo Effect: Predictions From the Model. In L. White, B. Tursky, and G. E. Schwartz, eds., *Placebo: Theory, Research, and Mechanisms.* New York: Guilford Press.

The Role of Conditioning in Pharmacotherapy

Robert Ader

Introduction

When a physician gives you a pill, a salve, or an injection that contains no ingredients known to influence your cold symptoms, your rash, or your pain—but you experience relief from whatever it is that ails you, anyway—that is the "placebo effect." Shapiro (Chapter 1) defines the placebo effect as "the nonspecific, psychological, or psychophysiologic therapeutic effect produced by a placebo . . ." Descriptions of the placebo effect typically have had a pejorative quality; and even in the corridors of our medical institutions today, the "placebo effect" can be heard to refer to any effect for which we have no mechanistic explanation—a phenomenon that is not real.

There has been relatively little systematic exploration of the scope of placebo phenomena, a fact that may reflect the lack of any theoretical position(s) within which to organize existing data and upon which to base the design of new research. For the most part, clinical research and drug evaluation studies have adhered to the model in which a drug or placebo is administered in order to evaluate the efficacy of pharmacotherapies or to define the pharmacologic (as opposed to the psychologic) action of a drug. Thus, research has been directed to characterizations of the placebo itself; characterizations of beliefs and expectancies, including those induced by the instructions to subjects; and characterizations of the subjects who respond to placebos. These and similar variables—and the control conditions that are imposed in

138

drug research—derive, primarily, from an effort to define the "true," unadulterated action of a drug rather than an effort to understand the nature of the placebo effect and its therapeutic effects. Although there have been repeated calls for studies of the placebo effect as a phenomenon that may have clinical implications in its own right, there are still relatively few studies of this kind. This chapter will elaborate on a view of placebo effects that addresses the therapeutic potential of this component of drug treatment protocols.

Drugs do not act in a vacuum; they are superimposed upon behaving organisms. Therefore, the biologically relevant effects of drugs depend to a large extent on the interaction between the pharmacologic action of the drug and the psychobiologic state of the individual into whom it is introduced. That psychobiologic state is influenced by a myriad of variables from the genetic to the environmental. Some of the most immediate factors are daily rhythms, the emotional and motivational state of the individual, the individual's expectations, and the individual's experiential history with drugs, and, perhaps, other medical procedures. This chapter emphasizes the experiential drug history of the individual.

I accept but am not immediately concerned with the experiential history of the individual as a variable which, like any number of other variables, is capable of modulating the magnitude, duration, or even the direction of the initial response to a placebo. And it is the initial response to a placebo, whether in experimental subjects or patients, that is studied in the vast majority of the research on placebo effects. I am interested in a malleable experiential history that can contribute clinical import to current conceptualizations of placebo effects. I am quite aware that one cannot, with impunity, attempt to redefine a cherished concept, however inadequate or confusing the current concept is or may become. Some definitions of the placebo effect, for example, include a phrase that presumes the means by which the effect occurs. Thus, the placebo effect may, by definition, be due to the patient's belief (or faith or expectations) that relief will be forthcoming. If such assumptions are accepted as part of the definition of the placebo effect, I will not be speaking about the placebo effect. If the placebo effect is, by definition, a *nonspecific* effect, I will not be speaking about the placebo effect. I will be speaking about some other phenomenon—a placebo effect, perhaps—which, for want of an appropriate label, deals with the role of conditioning in pharmacotherapy. Nevertheless, some have found it interesting, provocative, or inescapable that the role of conditioning in pharmacotherapy be presented within the context of a discussion of the placebo effect. This situation may be particularly appropriate for a volume in which participants were invited to create some destabilization of current thinking with respect to placebo effects.

I will, then, discuss the role of conditioning in pharmacotherapeutic regimens. The reader will decide how this bears on or modifies current conceptualizations and approaches to an understanding of placebo effects, experimental and clinical approaches to the evaluation of drugs, and the design of treatment protocols—and the reader's vote will be cast in the research that is undertaken.

The Placebo Effect as a Conditioned Response

The response to a placebo "looks like" the response to a conditioned stimulus (CS). In behavioral terms, the physiological effects unconditionally elicited by pharmacologic agents are unconditioned responses (UCRs), the drug itself being the unconditioned stimulus (UCS). The environmental or behavioral events or stimuli that are coincidentally or purposely associated with and reliably precede the voluntary or involuntary receipt of drug—but that are neutral with respect to eliciting the unconditioned effects of the active drug—are conditioned stimuli (CSs). These could include the bottle containing the drug; the room, or its color or smell, in which medication is taken or where it is administered (and by whom); and the "pill" or injection itself. The repeated association of CS and UCS eventually enables the CS to elicit a conditioned response (CR)—an approximation of the response unconditionally elicited by the UCS. Thus, the response to an inert or therapeutically irrelevant substance or placebo has been described as a conditioned response.

The notion that a placebo is a conditioned stimulus is not new. The placebo effect has been likened to a conditioned response or, at least, the influence of learning on the response to a placebo has been considered by several investigators (Wolf 1950; Skinner 1953; Stanley and

Schlosberg 1953; Lasagna et al. 1954; Gleidman, Gantt, and Teitelbaum 1957; Kurland 1957; Beecher 1959; Petrie 1960; Herrnstein 1962; Knowles 1963; Ross and Schnitzer 1963; Pihl and Altman 1971; Wikler 1973; Evans 1974; Voudouris, Peck, and Coleman 1985; Gadow, White, and Ferguson 1985). One of the more denotative descriptions of the placebo effect as a CR has been provided by Wickramesekera (1980) who, like others, argues that the entire ritual surrounding drug treatment can become a CS by virtue of the repeated association of such neutral cues with active drug administration in the history of the patient.

Several experiments have specifically addressed the placebo effect as a conditioning phenomenon. Most of these have been conducted in animals (Herrnstein 1962; Ross and Schnitzer 1963; Lang, Ross, and Glover 1967; Pihl and Altman 1971; Roffman, Reddy, and Lal 1973; Deutsch 1974; Numan, Smith, and Lal 1975; Hayshi, Ohashi, and Takadoro 1980); but a few experiments have been conducted with humans (Voudouris, Peck, and Coleman 1985; Zwyghuizen-Doorenbos et al. 1990; Suchman and Ader 1992). Zwyghuizen-Doorenbos and her colleagues examined the conditioning of the alerting effects of caffeine, and Voudouris and his colleagues reported that conditioning could attenuate or exacerbate the response to experimentally induced pain stimulation.

In animals, Herrnstein (1962) found that, under appropriate temporal conditions, rats would respond to an injection of saline with a suppression of the behavioral reactions that characterized their previous responses to scopolamine hydrobromide. Similarly, after one or more injections of d-amphetamine, the unconditioned increase in activity could be observed after an injection of saline, and it was noted that the magnitude of the placebo response was a function of the number of times the active drug had previously been injected (Pihl and Altman 1971; Ross and Schnitzer 1963). Pavlov (1927) had described what appear to have been conditioned morphine effects, and both Roffman et al. (1973) and Numan et al. (1975) found that the repeated pairing of an auditory stimulus with injections of morphine enabled subsequent presentations of the tone alone to reduce the hypothermia and body shakes that accompany morphine withdrawal in the rat. Other recent observations implicate learning processes in the physiologic (immunologic) response to antigenic stimulation. Dolin and Krylov (1952) claimed that the repeated injection of rabbits with saline resulted in a conditioned depression in the antibody response to a subsequent injection of antigen. Shaskin and Lovett (1981) described a similar effect for a cell-mediated immune response, and Moynihan et al. (1989) also found that repeated ip injections of saline attenuated the antibody response to a subsequent ip injection of antigen in mice. Conversely, and with more extensive control conditions, when a CS was repeatedly paired with low dose injections of antigen, a classically conditioned enhancement of antibody production occurred when conditioned mice were reexposed to the CS in the context of reexposure to a minimally immunogenic dose of that same antigen (Ader et al. 1993).

There is, too, a voluminous literature on the conditioning of drug-induced physiological responses (Miller 1969; Harris and Brady 1974; Eikelboom and Stewart 1982) and its clinical implications, especially in relation to drug addiction (Lynch et al. 1973; Siegel 1983). These data on conditioned pharmacologic responses bear on the notion of the placebo effect being a conditioned response; however, as I will suggest later, they may not prove to be the most immediately relevant data upon which to base an analysis of placebo effects.

In view of the existing data, then, the proposition that the placebo effect is a conditioned response is not new. It is surprising, though, that few investigators have attempted a systematic analysis of the placebo effect within the context of conditioning. The notion of the placebo effect as a conditioned response has, for all practical purposes, remained at a descriptive level and has not generated research strategies designed to evaluate the hypothesis or test the predictions that would follow from such an analysis: the response to a placebo "looks like" the response to a conditioned stimulus.

The Role of Conditioning in Pharmacotherapies

If the placebo effect is a conditioned response, what are the therapeutic implications, and what are the implications for psychopharmacologic research? Currently, research designed to evaluate drug effects involves only two groups: an experimental group that receives active drug and a control group that does not, receiving instead an inert or chemically irrelevant substance (the placebo). In all other respects, the stimuli that attend drug or placebo administration are, theoretically, "identical." No matter how the dose, route of administration, frequency, or duration of treatment may be varied, experimental subjects receive medication that is invariably followed (reinforced) by the unconditioned effects of the drug (a continuous or 100 percent reinforcement schedule). In contrast, control subjects who engage in the same behaviors are subject to the same environmental conditions, and they receive placebo medication that are never therapeutically reinforced; the control subjects are on a 0 percent reinforcement schedule. One is therefore prompted to ask, "What about schedules of reinforcement between 0 and 100 percent?"

There is, evidently, an alternative to evaluating drug effects by administering drug *or* placebo: one can administer drug *and* placebo. That is, one can introduce partial schedules of reinforcement in which "medication" and the attendant environmental cues are pharmacologically reinforced on some occasions but not on others. Schedule of reinforcement, the "active drug:placebo ratio," in other words, becomes another means for titrating cumulative drug dose. Instead of lowering the concentration of drug received whenever drug is administered, cumulative drug dose could be lowered under a long-term regimen of pharmacotherapy by prescribing a 90 percent, 75 percent, or 50 percent schedule of reinforcement in which only 90 percent, 75 percent, or 50 percent of the medication received would actually contain active drug; for the remainder of the time the patient would be receiving inert medication—CSs that have, in the past, been invariably associated with the unconditional effects of the active medication. By capitalizing on conditioning effects, it might be possible to approximate the therapeutic effects of a continuous schedule of pharmacologic reinforcement, that is, to relieve pain or maintain some physiologic state within homeostatic limits, using lower cumulative amounts of drug.

Despite the suggestions (Herrnstein 1962; Evans 1974) and some clinical data (Greenberg and Roth 1966), there have been few if any studies in which drug and placebo have been interspersed, and no studies that have systematically varied the schedule of pharmacologic reinforcement in examining the efficacy of different therapeutic regimens. There are, however, several observations that are relevant to this conditioning interpretation of the placebo effect.

Pharmacotherapy Studies

Pairing a neutral CS with cyclophosphamide, an immunosuppressive drug, enables the CS to attenuate antibody- and cell-mediated immune responses when conditioned animals are subsequently immunized and reexposed to the CS alone (Ader and Cohen 1993). In an effort to elaborate the biologic impact of conditioned immunosuppressive responses, Ader and Cohen (1982) applied conditioning operations to the pharmacotherapy of autoimmune disease in female New Zealand hybrid mice genetically prone to the development of a lupus-like disorder.

One group of animals experienced a "standard" pharmacotherapeutic regimen: weekly pairings of saccharin (CS) and cyclophosphamide (CY), the UCS—a continuous schedule of pharmacologic reinforcement. A second group of conditioned animals was treated on a 50 percent reinforcement schedule. These mice were exposed to saccharin and ip injections weekly, but they received CY on only half the trials. The development of proteinuria and mortality was significantly delayed in these mice relative to an untreated group and, more importantly, relative to a nonconditioned group that received the same number of exposures to saccharin and CY, but in an unpaired (noncontingent) manner. There were no differences between these latter two groups. Thus, exposure to the CS paired with active drug (placebo treatments) potentiated the effects of a treatment regimen that was insufficient, by itself, to alter the course of the autoimmune disease.

In a separate experiment (Ader 1985), lupus-prone mice that had been treated with saccharin and CY for two and a half months were divided into three subgroups: one subgroup continued to receive CS-UCS pairings; another continued to receive weekly exposures to the CS followed by an injection of saline rather than CY; and a third subgroup received neither saccharin nor CY. Pharmacologically, the latter two subgroups were the same; neither received any active drug therapy. Mice that continued to be reexposed to the CS survived significantly longer than the conditioned group that experienced neither the drug nor the CS. In fact, animals that continued to be exposed to the CS did not differ from animals that continued to receive active drug. Reexposure to saccharin had no effect on nonconditioned animals; these mice did not differ from those for whom both the CS and UCS were discontinued. Such findings suggested that there might be considerable heuristic value in viewing a pharmacotherapeutic regimen as a series of conditioning trials and in adopting a conditioning model for manipulating, controlling, and predicting placebo effects in pharmacotherapeutic situations.

A clinical case study of a child with lupus (Olness and Ader 1992) was based specifically on these observations. During the course of twelve months, a clinically successful outcome was achieved by providing only the CSs on half the monthly chemotherapy sessions. There are few definitive conclusions to be drawn from a single case report; however, considering the toxic effects of cytoxan, these are intriguing observations that would seem to justify additional clinical studies in selected patients requiring immunosuppressive therapy.

A study of inpatient schizophrenics (Greenberg and Roth 1966) also yielded positive results. In an attempt to reduce the amount of tranquilizing drug given to hospitalized schizophrenics on a daily basis, the amount of chlorpromazine was reduced by substituting a placebo for active drug on one day of each week. There were no untoward effects, so a regimen of drug on five days and placebo on two days was introduced, and one additional "placebo day" was added every eight weeks. The gradual reduction of the schedule of pharmacologic reinforcement was successful in the maintenance of this population of schizophrenics, many of whom were treated with chlorpromazine only two or three times per week. Although conditioning processes could have been responsible for this effect, the design of the study, which was not intended to assess conditioning effects, does not permit one to draw that conclusion. The conclusion that schizophrenics may be receiving more medication than necessary may also be true but does not follow from these data. It is possible that these schizophrenic patients could be maintained on medication two or three days per week only because they received placebo medication (CSs) and experienced conditioned drug effects on the remaining days. Assuming that a given drug dose does not exceed some threshold level, receiving active drug x days each week and inactive drug y days each week is pharmacologically equivalent to receiving only active drug x days each week. Psychopharmacologically, however, these may be very different treatment regimens that have very different long-term effects. That possibility remains to be tested.

Sequence Effects

If learning processes were not involved in placebo effects—that is, if the placebo effect were simply attributable to faith in the system or in one's physician, or perhaps to a function of some personal characteristic—one would expect that one placebo would be as effective as another and that a placebo would be equally effective no matter when it was administered. However, experimental and clinical data clearly indicate that there is a greater placebo effect when placebo medication is given after a period of effective drug treatment than when it is given as the "first" medication.

Among patients receiving drugs for the relief of musculoskeletal pain, Batterman (1966) found that a significant number of patients who were switched from drug to placebo remained free of pain long after the "die-away" time of the drug's effect. Sunshine et al. (1964) also reported that, as an initial response to medication, aspirin and indomethacin were more effective in relieving pain than placebo. As a second or third medication, however, there were no differences between the active drugs and placebo. Similar results were reported by Moertel et al. (1976). Earlier, Batterman (1965) showed that not only was placebo medication more effective when it followed active and effective drug therapy but that active drug was less effective when it followed an ineffective period of treatment relative to its effectiveness as a first medication or when it followed other effective medication.

In this regard, it is of some interest that Prien et al. (1968) have noted that, although the data on tranquilizers are not uniform, studies in which schizophrenic patients have been taken off drug and provided with no medication report a higher incidence and more rapid rate of relapse than studies in which active medication is replaced by a placebo.

Crossover Designs

The most prominent example of a sequence effect is the purportedly ubiquitous observation that when subjects or patients are switched from a regimen of active drug treatment to a period of placebo treatment, the physiologic levels and/or clinical symptoms for which the drug was administered do not immediately return to the pretreatment baseline. Among those who are given placebo following initial treatment with active drug in a crossover design (Figure 7.1), the effects of the drug can persist for a period of time that exceeds the known residual effects of the drug. No satisfactory explanation has been given for this "asymmetry" in the curves representing the functional effects of drug and placebo in a crossover study of drug effects.

Several explanations have been offered for such findings (Batterman 1966): (a) the findings could reflect the behavior of placebo "reactors"; (b) there may have been spontaneous cessation of the original complaints; (c) in a clinical setting, specific actions of the drug may have corrected the precipitating condition and so therapy may no longer have been needed; (d) effective drugs could influence the response to subsequent drugs, and the observed effects were due to the patients' expectations (conditioning); (e) and—the possibility favored—some drugs may exert effects that persist beyond their presence in the body by influencing enzyme systems or receptor sites that require time to recover normal function. Possibility (e) is a parsimonious hypothesis. Nonetheless, the observation of prolonged effects when inactive drug follows active (and effective) drug treatment is exactly what one would predict if conditioning occurred during the period of active pharmacotherapy. That is, having repeatedly experienced the pairing of a number of constant stimuli, including the pill containing the active drug (the CSs), with the effects unconditionally elicited by the active drug, reexposure to the CS alone was capable of evoking the same or similar reactions.

With respect to the hypothesis that the residual drug effects extended the effects of medication after discontinuation of treatment, neither direct nor indirect residual effects of an active drug can be defined in the presence of placebo medication. A functional definition of the residual effects of a given concentration of drug administered at a given frequency and for a given duration of time can be defined only by individuals for whom active drug treatment is followed by a period of "no medication." Such a group is not included in the classic crossover design. Therefore, to the extent that it is important to document

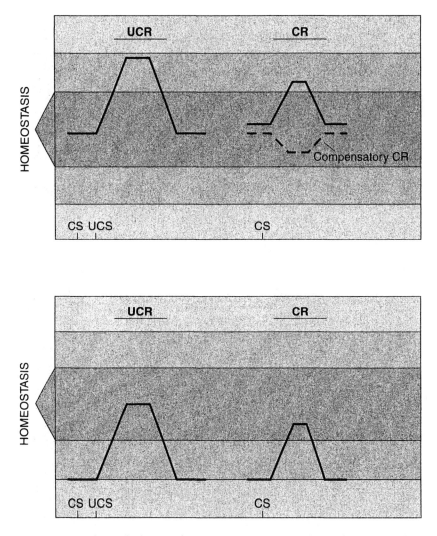

Figure 7.1 Conditioned pharmacologic response *(top)*. Conditioned pharmacothera-peutic response *(bottom)*.

residual drug effects and/or understand placebo effects *within* rather than *between* individuals, the crossover design is incomplete.

In addition to quantifying direct or indirect residual drug effects, a "no medication" control group enables one to assess the magnitude of the placebo effect—or the effects of conditioning. Pharmacologically, there should be no difference between a "no medication" group and a "placebo" group since neither group receives active drug. However, during a period of active drug therapy, patients are learning the relationship between environmental cues and the physiologic and therapeutic consequences of a drug. One would predict, then, that conditioned physiologic and therapeutic effects would occur and that, phenomenologically (and practically), the effects of prior drug treatment would persist longer in the "placebo" (CS reexposure) group than in the "no medication" (no CS reexposure) group. Hypothetically, the difference might approximate that shown schematically in Figure 7.1. Furthermore, if conditioning occurs during the period of pharmacotherapy, one would predict that, following the discontinuation of active drug treatment, the duration of the drug effect among individuals reexposed to CSs would be a function of the schedule of reinforcement that was in effect during the period of pharmacotherapy.

Precipitated by this analysis of crossover effects, Götestam et al. (1995) reassessed the results of a study by Hogarty et al. (1973) comparing one-year relapse rates of schizophrenics maintained on drug or placebo following discharge from the hospital. For those who continued to take active drug, the relapse rate was 16.8 percent; and for those taking placebo medication, the relapse rate was 53.1 percent. But for those patients who did not take their placebo medication, the relapse rate was 74.7 percent; and for those who, at some point, stopped taking their active drug, the relapse rate was 61.2 percent. Although there was no experimental "no medication" group—and these results are confounded by the time at which patients stopped taking medication—the findings are consistent with those of Prien et al. (1968) and with the hypothesized effects of conditioning during the previous period of inpatient drug therapy.

In a recent study (Suchman and Ader 1992), these hypothetical results were observed in patients being treated with atenolol for essential hypertension. Patients who were treated with a placebo following active medication maintained normotensive blood pressure levels significantly longer than patients who were first treated with atenolol and then given no medication. The latter group defined the residual effects of these doses of atenolol, and, in the absence of active drug, the effects of continued exposure to the CSs exceeded these residual drug effects—a (psychopharmacologic) effect for which there is no pharmacologic explanation. These results are quite consistent, but they provide no direct evidence that conditioning occurred during the initial period of pharmacotherapy.

If this analysis of crossover effects is correct, it has further methodological implications. Periods of time during which no drugs are administered ("wash out" periods) are frequently imposed in an effort to "start from scratch," so to speak, before a first therapeutic drug is administered, either before repeating a regimen of drug administration or before introducing a different drug. Wash-out periods may eliminate the presence or effects of prior drug(s), but they cannot eliminate a learned response. Thus, patients or experimental subjects return to a regimen of drug administration with the conditioned response acquired under the prior period of drug administration intact. Unless the "wash-out" period is a lot longer than could probably be tolerated in clinical situations or experimental protocols, the effects of conditioning can be eliminated only by extinguishing the conditioned response, that is, by presenting the CS without the UCS.

Side Effects

Would not the conditioning of pharmacotherapeutic effects also result in the conditioning of side effects? Probably so. Among cancer patients being treated with analgesics for pain relief, those who responded to placebo had the greater response rate to active drug, and they had the higher incidence of CNS-mediated side effects to placebo (Moertel et al. 1976).

Drugs have multiple effects, some of which are sometimes called side or secondary effects depending on the interests of the investigator. Although such effects are not necessarily injurious or even unpleasant, the question addresses the benefit to be gained from drug-induced conditioned responses. By definition, such conditioned side effects could not be more prevalent or intense than the unconditioned side effects elicited by the continuous administration of active drug. In fact, any deleterious side effects elicited by the direct action of the medication would, in a conditioning model, be less prevalent because there would be fewer administrations of active drug among patients treated under a partial schedule of pharmacologic reinforcement.

One major concern in drug research has been the extent to which subjects or patients and experimenters are truly "blinded" (Ney, Collins, and Spensor 1986; Moscucci et al. 1987; Bystritsky and Waikar 1994). As one might suppose, humans use whatever cues may be available to guess whether they are receiving active or inactive medication; and the guessing can be quite accurate depending upon the effects of the medication (sometimes it is the placebo and sometimes the drug condition that is correctly identified). (Parenthetically, more attention has been paid to calculating the accuracy of guesses than to the impact of correct and incorrect guesses.) Primary among the cues used by subjects and experimenters is the presence or absence of side effects. Using "active" placebos can be effective, but, ideally, some protocols such as those involving chronic drug treatment and changes in reinforcement schedule would require reproducing side effects elicited by the active drug under study. Thus, it can be very difficult to have a perfect placebo—especially since drug effects, primary or secondary, are different in different individuals. Under these circumstances, conditioned side effects would increase the similarity between drug and placebo conditions and amplify placebo effects (Thomson 1982).

Compensatory Conditioned Responses

Conditioned pharmacologic effects are sometimes in a direction opposite to the responses elicited by the drug used as the UCS. Drugs that act on the afferent or input arm of the CNS yield CRs that mimic the unconditioned effects of the drug. Drugs that act on the efferent arm of the CNS, that is, have a direct effect on some target organ, elicit a response that appears to be opposite in direction from the ostensible UCR. As argued by Eichelboom and Stewart (1982) and Miller and Dworkin (1980), it is the target organ response that provides the afferent signal to the CNS and constitutes the UCS for a response that is opposite in direction to and compensates for the target organ change. One of the more notable illustrations of such effects involves the role of conditioning in the development of tolerance to some drugs (Siegel 1983). Predicting the direction of drug-induced conditioned physiologic and, presumably, pharmacotherapeutic effects, therefore, would depend upon knowledge of the site(s) of action of the pharmacologic agent. But, it seems, that is so neither all the time nor under all conditions.

In experimental studies with animals, reproducing the environmental context in which morphine is administered yields hyperalgesia (Siegel 1983); reexposing animals to a gustatory stimulus paired with morphine administration, however, elicits an analgesic response upon reexposure to the gustatory CS (Miller et al. 1990). With respect to the effects of morphine on body temperature, some studies report a compensatory hypothermic conditioned response (tolerance), while several others (Sherman 1979) describe a conditioned hyperthermic response. Thus, these and other data on conditioned insulin (Storlien et al. 1985) or conditioned hypotensive drug effects (Lang et al. 1967) indicate that the site of action of the drug does not alone determine the direction of the conditioned response.

Other seemingly contradictory findings are results from analyses of previously conducted crossover studies suggesting that the more effective the tranquilizer, the weaker the placebo response (Rickels et al. 1966). Although the results are quite variable, data on schizophrenics indicate that the withdrawal of medication and substitution of a placebo is associated with a lower rate of relapse than the discontinuation of medication without providing a placebo (Prien et al. 1968). In their own analysis of data obtained from seven hospitals, Prien and his associates found that, within the group given placebo following the discontinuation of phenothiazines, relapse was directly related to the dose of the patients' prior medication. There were, however, large differences in the data obtained from different hospitals. Whether such findings could reflect the conditioning of compensatory responses (see Chapter 8) or, in this instance, the ease of discrimination between the effects of active drug and placebo (the use of an active or inactive placebo is not specified) is not clear. There is, of course, the additional possibility that medication dose was determined by severity of symptoms so that relapse rate was, in fact, related to the degree of disturbance of the patients. In any case, the opposite is true of analgesics: the more effective the prior medication has been, the greater the magnitude or duration of the placebo effect (Kantor et al. 1966; Batterman and Lower 1968; Laska and Sunshine 1973; Moertel et al. 1976; Voudouris et al. 1985). One explanation of such apparent inconsistencies is that the expectancy of analgesia (in humans) overrides the compensatory response that can be produced by conditioning (in rats) (Kirsch, Chapter 8). There is no evidence here of compensatory conditioning, and such an effect seems unlikely considering the observed dose-response effect. It can be difficult to establish any generalizable relationships from studies of human patients suffering from pain who are treated with placebos and healthy rats that are given analgesics and then subjected to experimentally induced pain. Also, these and other data make it evident that no single model (such as analgesia) or no single class of drugs (such as tranquilizers) can be taken as *the* model for assessing or understanding the placebo effect.

Conditioned Pharmacologic and Pharmacotherapeutic Responses

The psychophysiologic state of the subject or patient is an especially critical variable that might influence the direction of the effects of conditioning. Taking this into consideration, it can be argued that the literature on conditioned pharmacologic responses is relevant but not critical to an analysis of the placebo effect as a conditioned response and the role of conditioning in pharmacotherapies. In fact, a concentration on the conditioning of pharmacologic responses and its relation to the initial response to a placebo actually confuses a discussion of the therapeutic implications to be derived from a recognition of the role of conditioning in drug treatment regimens.

Operationally, there is a major difference between conditioned *pharmacologic* responses and conditioned *pharmacotherapeutic* responses. In conditioning pharmacologic response(s), normal (healthy) human or nonhuman subjects are brought into a laboratory where they are exposed to one or more pairings of a neutral CS and the pharmacologic agent that unconditionally elicits one or more quantifiable physiological responses. Subsequent presentation of the CS alone elicits a conditioned response which may mimic in direction and approach in magnitude the physiological effect(s) induced by the UCS. Under certain circumstances and in the case of certain drugs, the response elicited by the CS is opposite in direction to that evoked by the UCS. This so-called paradoxical or compensatory conditioned response is presumed to occur in anticipation of and as a means of attenuating the effects of the UCS—a mechanism calculated to assure that the unconditioned response does not exceed homeostatic limits that could threaten the integrity of the organism.

In contrast, a conditioned pharmacotherapeutic response involves exposing "patients" or, perhaps, a species of animal—animals that spontaneously develop a particular disease or in which a dysregulated physiological state has been induced experimentally—to one or more pairings of a neutral CS and a pharmacologic agent that unconditionally elicits one or more physiological responses calculated to correct the naturally occurring or experimentally induced physiologic imbalance. Thus, the study of conditioned pharmacologic responses involves an analysis of responses that deviate from a normal baseline or that might prevent a deviation from homeostasis, whereas the study of conditioned pharmacotherapeutic responses involves responses designed to restore or maintain homeostasis. In the latter case, a compensatory CR could exacerbate the preexisting physiologic dysregulation to the detriment of the organism. Teleologically, such an outcome would violate the so-called "wisdom of the body" and negate the interpretation of learning as a mechanism that serves adaptive ends.

This basic and, perhaps, critical difference between conditioned pharmacologic and pharmacotherapeutic responses is schematized in Figure 7.2. It cannot be assumed that precisely the same functional relationships among conditioning variables would apply in each of these cases. Indeed, there are grounds for hypothesizing that the mechanisms underlying conditioned pharmacologic and pharmacotherapeutic effects may be different. That the same drugs which induce compensatory conditioned responses in normal, healthy subjects would not induce compensatory responses in subjects for whom that drug was therapeutic is a testable hypothesis. Existing data on taste aversions and taste preferences for substances that either cause or correct homeostatic disturbances (Rozin and Kalat 1971), for example, illustrate that what is learned is very much dependent on the state of the organism. This event appears to occur even in the case of the purportedly autonomous immune system. Normal mice acquire conditioned taste aversions to gustatory stimuli associated with the effects of lithium chloride (LiCl) or cyclophosphamide (CY); however, although lupus-prone mice are capable of acquiring an aversion based on LiCl, they do not, depending on dose, display a taste aversion

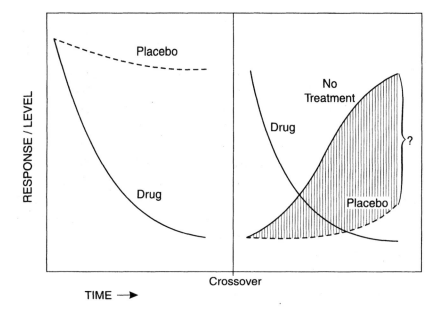

Figure 7.2 Difference between conditioned pharmacologic and pharmacotherapeutic responses

based on CY, an immunosuppressive drug that promotes their survival (Ader et al. 1991).

Applications and Implications of a Conditioning Model of Pharmacotherapy

Conceptualizing a pharmacotherapeutic regimen as a series of conditioning trials suggests new strategies for assessing drug and placebo effects and testable hypotheses that derive from a learning perspective. Prominent among these strategies would be the institution of different schedules of pharmacologic reinforcement. Employing the proposition that conditioning takes place during some pharmacotherapies, one can describe a variation of the pharmacologic reinforcement schedule as a variation of the "active drug:placebo ratio" which, like the dose, route, frequency, and duration of medication, is an additional dimension of a pharmacotherapeutic regimen and an alternative means for adjusting cumulative drug dose. Under a prolonged regimen of pharmacotherapy, cumulative drug dose might be lowered, not by gradually lowering the concentration of drug administered on each of the component drug trials but rather by gradually lowering the reinforcement schedule. One could not expect conditioning to occur in those situations in which drugs are prescribed to replace what a target organ is unable to produce. However, this option, which capitalizes on conditioned physiologic effects, leads to testable predictions regarding the effects of placebo medication that, if confirmed, suggest new strategies for psychopharmacologic research. The option also suggests strategies for a new combination of behavioral and pharmacologic interventions designed to regulate a variety of other physiological processes.

For patients maintained on long-term pharmacotherapeutic regimens, especially in the case of drugs with noxious or deleterious "side effects" such as adrenal steroids or other immunosuppressive agents, the prescription of partial schedules of drug reinforcement might reduce the total amount of drug required to treat some pathophysiological condition or maintain some physiologic state within homeostatic limits. It cannot be known, a priori what schedule of reinforcement to impose. Therefore, a conservative beginning would be to reduce the reinforcement schedule in patients who are stable under a continuous schedule of reinforcement—a clinical situation that might now prompt a reduction in the concentration of drug prescribed. Indeed, any clinical study in which the schedule of reinforcement was reduced (gradually within subjects, or with different reinforcement schedules in different groups) will require comparison groups that receive the same (reduced) cumulative amount of drug under a continuous schedule of reinforcement. That is, patients under a 75 percent reinforcement schedule would receive their full dose of active drug 75 percent of the time (a placebo would be administered 25 percent of the time). A second experimental group would remain under a 100 percent reinforcement schedule, but the concentration of drug would be reduced to 75 percent of the original dose. Eventually, it is conceivable that only an occasional reinforcement would be required to maintain the clinical effectiveness of the placebo.

Conversely, under conditions in which the clinician might want to increase the dose of medication but is constrained by toxic target organ effects, an ostensible increase in the amount of drug being taken might be achieved by keeping the dose constant but using placebos to increase the number of occasions per day or per week on which medication would be taken. Still another variation of the theme can be derived from the study on conditioned enhancement of antibody production (Ader et al. 1993). Neither the CS alone nor a low-dose booster injection of antigen was sufficient to elevate antibody titers, but, in the presence of the booster dose of antigen, reexposure to the CS enhanced antibody production. In a drug treatment protocol, there could be situations in which one might want to consider a "partial" schedule of reinforcement in which the CS-only trials actually consisted of the CS containing a low, ineffective, or minimally effective dose of the active drug.

Treatment under a partial schedule of drug reinforcement is likely to reduce the magnitude of side effects because CRs are not typically as large as UCRs. If side effects are reduced, adherence to the treatment protocol may increase. Clinically, this situation is to be desired; experimentally, it poses an additional problem: patients under a partial schedule of reinforcement may actually take more of their medication than they did under a continuous schedule of reinforcement, so adherence to the treatment protocol needs to be monitored. The fact that less active drug is present could also have consequences for target organ damage and, conceivably, for addressing problems of drug dependence and drug withdrawal.

Theoretically, a partial schedule of reinforcement should extend the effects of pharmacotherapy, that is, increase resistance to experimental extinction. The "partial reinforcement effect" refers to observations that resistance to extinction is greater for responses acquired under partial reinforcement than under continuous reinforcement. It was once thought that the partial reinforcement effect did not obtain in classical conditioning. However, Mackintosh (1974), for one, has argued that the available data provide no grounds for distinguishing between classical and instrumental conditioning on this basis; and also the effect has been observed in classical conditioning studies with different species performing different responses to different CSs and UCSs (Farrell et al. 1980). In one study (Gibbs et al. 1976), partial schedules of reinforcement were introduced after the response in question had been acquired under a continuous schedule of reinforcement (a strategy recommended for the maintenance of conditioned pharmacotherapeutic responses). Extinction was relatively rapid in animals that remained on a continuous reinforcement schedule, but the response level remained high even among animals that had been reduced to a 15 percent reinforcement schedule. Further, the distinction between classical and instrumental conditioning is itself blurred, and conditioned pharmacotherapeutic responses represent a situation in which, for a conscious individual, the UCS can never be introduced in the absence of CSs and in which there are elements of both classical and instrumental conditioning. Therefore, it is predicted that continued presentation of CSs (placebo) after active drug is discontinued would extend the effects of active drug for a longer period of time among patients treated with the same cumulative amount of drug under a partial than under a continuous schedule of pharmacologic reinforcement. If this turns out to be the case, this strategy might profitably be applied in attempting to wean patients from certain drugs.

The maintenance of patients under a partial schedule of pharmacologic reinforcement might also influence the interaction between pharmacotherapeutic and psychotherapeutic interventions. In psychiatric patients, for example, such a treatment regimen might enable psychotherapeutic interventions to be conducted during symptom-free periods that were not completely regulated by the continuous presence of drug. If the phenomenon of state-dependent learning were utilized, the coping behaviors learned under these conditions might be more readily generalized and might facilitate the ultimate transition to a drug-free state.

As an ethical issue with additional implications for informed consent and for the instructions given to subjects or patients, the institution of conditioning operations would obviate the need for a "no treatment" group in some clinical research. Systematic variation of reinforcement schedule would define a functional relationship between the "active drug:placebo ratio" (or cumulative dose) and outcome that would not be meaningfully enhanced by the data from a zero reinforcement group. (Systematic variation might also increase the number of volunteers willing to participate in testing the efficacy of new drugs.)

Finally, if capitalizing on conditioned pharmacotherapeutic responses enabled patients to be maintained on a partial schedule of pharmacologic reinforcement that approximated the therapeutic effects of "standard treatment"—a continuous schedule of reinforcement—one would be maximizing the benefits, minimizing the risks, and reducing substantially the cost of long-term drug treatment.

Conclusion

The lack of scientific attention devoted to the placebo effect as a phenomenon in its own right probably reflects the paucity of theoretical positions within which to organize the existing data and upon which to base the design of new research. The arguments presented here are an attempt to advance from a descriptive to an experimental analysis of the placebo effect as a reflection of learning processes and to examine the clinical implications of such an analysis.

It was not my intent to redefine "the placebo effect," but rather my intent was to provoke a reexamination of the scope of placebo phenomena. The placebo effect has never been studied as an inseparable component of a regimen of pharmacotherapy. However, with the exception of replacement therapies, all pharmacotherapeutic regimens contain within them an element of conditioning. Operationally, it is not possible to administer a drug for therapeutic purposes that is not accompanied by conditioned stimuli. However, conditioned stimuli do not have to be labelled "placebos." In a sense, the present analysis does not consider the placebo effect in a new context as much as it looks at the conditioning component of pharmacotherapies and, looking back, seems to impose that definition of a placebo onto the phenomena that have been studied thus far. One could even take the position that a conditioned stimulus cannot be a placebo if a placebo is, by definition, neutral with respect to the physiologic changes induced by the therapeutic agent. A conditioned stimulus is neutral only the first time that it is presented; once it has been paired with an unconditioned stimulus, it is no longer neutral!

There is, I believe, considerable heuristic value in viewing a pharmacotherapeutic regimen as a series of conditioning trials. Whether this is *the* placebo effect or *a* placebo effect—or whether the effects of manipulating conditioning variables in a pharmacotherapeutic regimen even apply in nontherapeutic situations—remains to be determined.

How the differences between therapeutic and nontherapeutic settings are understood and how the implicit specificity of conditioned responses relate to apparent contradictions in the placebo literature also remain to be determined. In any case, the label is not important; it does not alter the strategies that do apply in attempting to capitalize on conditioned pharmacotherapeutic responses. Of course, one can choose to ignore the conditioning component of pharmacotherapies. Alternatively, one can explore ways in which to exploit this conditioning in designing drug treatment regimens that consider both the behavioral and the pharmacologic components of the response to drugs.

Whether or not the model proposed turns out to have any merit, the adoption of a conditioning perspective suggests testable hypotheses and innovative strategies for the experimental analysis of drug and placebo effects and for the design of pharmacotherapeutic regimens. One of the advantages of adopting a conditioning perspective in the evaluation and application of pharmacotherapeutic regimens would include the availability of animal models of disease within which to examine conditioning effects. Clinical research findings could have a profound impact on the design of pharmacotherapeutic regimens. Central among these would be the possibility of achieving short- and long-term therapeutic goals using lower maintenance levels of drugs that would maximize the benefits and that would, in many instances, reduce the risks of prescribing certain drugs for certain clinical disorders. Should this be the case, the reduction in the costs of medication would not be insignificant.

References

Ader, R. 1985. "Conditioned Immunopharmacological Effects in Animals: Implications for a Conditioning Model of Pharmacotherapy." *Placebo: Theory, Research and Mechanisms.* New York: Guilford Press.

———— 1988. "The Placebo Effect as a Conditioned Response." *Experimental Foundations of Behavioral Medicine: Conditioning Approaches.* Hillside, N.J.: Lawrence Erlbaum.

———— 1989. "Conditioning Effects in Pharmacotherapy and the Incompleteness of the Double-Blind, Crossover Design." *Integrative Psychiatry,* 6:165–170.

Ader, R., and N. Cohen. 1982. "Behaviorally Conditioned Immunosuppression and Murine Systemic Lupus Erythematous." *Science,* 215:1534–1536.

—— 1993. "Psychoneuroimmunology: Conditioning and Stress." *Annual Review of Psychology,* 44:53–85.

Ader, R., L. J. Grota, J. A. Moynihan, and N. Cohen. 1991. "Behavioral Adaptations in Autoimmune Disease-Susceptible Mice." *Psychoneuroimmunology, Second Edition.* New York: Academic Press, p. 685–708.

Ader, R., K. Kelly, J. A. Moynihan, L. J. Grota, and N. Cohen. 1993. "Conditioned Enhancement of Antibody Production Using Antigen as the Unconditioned Stimulus." *Brain, Behavior, and Immunity,* 7:334–342.

Batterman, R. C. 1965. "Methodology of Analgesic Evaluation: Experience With Orphenadrine Citrate Compound." *Current Therapeutic Research,* 7:639–647.

—— 1966. "Persistence of Responsiveness With Placebo Therapy Following an Effective Drug Trial." *Journal of New Drugs,* 6:137–141.

Batterman, R. C., and W. R. Lower. 1968. "Placebo Responsiveness—Influence of Previous Therapy." *Current Therapeutic Research,* 10:136–143.

Beecher, H. K. 1959. *Measurement of Subjective Responses: Quantitative Effects of Drugs.* New York: Oxford University Press.

Bystritsky, A., and S. V. Waikar. 1994. "Inert Placebo Versus Active Medication: Patient Blindability in Clinical Pharmacological Trials." *Journal of Nervous and Mental Disease,* 182:485–487.

Deutsch, R. 1974. "Conditioned Hypoglycemia: A Mechanism for Saccharin-Induced Sensitivity to Insulin in the Rat." *Journal of Comparative and Physiological Psychology,* 86:350–358.

Dolin, A. O., and V. N. Krylov. 1952. "The Role of the Cerebral Cortex in Immune Reactions of the Organism." *Zhurnal Vysshei Nervnoi Deiatelnosti Imeni I. P. Pavlov,* 2:547–560.

Eikelboom, R., and J. Stewart. 1982. "Conditioning of Drug-Induced Physiological Responses." *Psychological Review,* 89:507–528.

Evans, F. J. 1974. "The Placebo Response in Pain Reduction." *Advances in Neurology,* 4:289–296.

Farrell, L., C., M. Locurto, H. J. Duncan, and H. S. Terrace. 1980. "Partial Reinforcement in Autoshaping with Pigeons." *Animal Learning and Behavior,* 8:45–59.

Gadow, K. D., and A. D. Poling. 1986. "Placebo Theory and Experimental Design." *Methodological Issues in Human Psychopharmacology: Advances in Learning and Behavioral Disabilities* (Supplement 1). Greenwich, Conn.: J. A. I. Press.

Gadow, K. D., L. White, and D. G. Ferguson. 1985. "Placebo Controls and Double-Blind Conditions." *Applied Psychopharmacology: Methods for Assessing Medication Effects.* New York: Grune and Stratton.

Gibbs, C. M., B. Latham, and I. Gormenzano. 1976. "Classical Conditioning of the Rabbit Nictitating Membrane Response: Effects of Reinforcement Schedule on Response Maintenance and Resistance to Extinction." *Animal Learning and Behavior*, 6:209–215.

Gleidman, L. H., W. H. Gantt, and H. A. Teitelbaum. 1957. "Some Implications of Conditional Reflex Studies for Placebo Research." *American Journal of Psychiatry*, 113:1103–1107.

Götestam, K. G., R. W. Gråwe, B. Lervåg, and J. H. Widén. 1995. "Does Placebo Give More Protection Against Relapse in Schizophrenia Than No Drug?" *European Journal of Psychiatry*, 9:58–62.

Greenberg, L. M., and S. Roth. 1966. "Differential Effects of Abrupt Versus Gradual Withdrawal of Chlorpromazine in Hospitalized Chronic Schizophrenic Patients." *American Journal of Psychiatry*, 123:221–226.

Harris, A. H., and J. V. Brady. 1974. "Animal Learning—Visceral and Autonomic Conditioning." *Annual Review of Psychology*, 25:107–133.

Hayashi, T., K. Ohashi, and S. Takadoro. 1980. "Conditioned Drug Effects to d-Amphetamine and Morphine-Induced Motor Acceleration in Mice: Experimental Approach for Placebo Effect." *Japanese Journal of Pharmacology*, 30:93–100.

Herrnstein, R. J. 1962. "Placebo Effect in the Rat." *Science*, 138:677–678.

Hogarty, G. E., S. C. Goldberg, and the Collaborative Study Group. 1973. "Drug and Sociotherapy in the Aftercare of Schizophrenic Patients." *Archives of General Psychiatry*, 28:54–64.

Kantor, T. G., A. Sunshine, E. Laskla, M. Meuisner, and M. Hopper. 1966. "Oral Analgesic Studies: Pentazocine Hydrochloride, Codeine, Aspirin, and Placebo and Their Influence on Response to Placebo." *Clinical Pharmacology and Therapeutics*, 7:447–454.

Knowles, J. B. 1963. "Conditioning and the Placebo Effect." *Behavioral Research*, 1:151–157.

Kurland, A. A. 1957. "The Drug Placebo: Its Psychodynamic and Conditioned Reflex Action." *Behavioral Science*, 2:101–110.

Lang, W. J., P. Ross, and A. Glover. 1967. "Conditional Response Induced by Hypotensive Drugs." *European Journal of Pharmacology*, 2:169–174.

Lasagna, L., F. Mosteller, J. M. von Pelsinger, and H. K. Beecher. 1954. "A Study of the Placebo Response." *American Journal of Medicine*, 16:770–779.

Laska, E., and A. Sunshine. 1973. "Anticipation of Analgesia—A Placebo Effect." *Headache*, 13:1–11.

Lynch, J. J., A. P. Fetziger, H. A. Teitelbaum, J. W. Cullen, and W. H. Gantt. 1973. "Pavlovian Conditioning of Drug Reactions: Some Implications for Problems of Drug Addiction." *Reflex*, 8:221–223.

Mackintosh, N. J. 1974. *The Psychology of Animal Learning*. New York: Academic Press.

Marlatt, G. A., and D. J. Rohsenow. 1980. "Cognitive Processes in Alcohol Use: Expectancy and the Balanced Placebo Design." *Advances in Substance Abuse,* 1:159–199.

Miller, J. S., K. S. Kelly, J. L. Neisewander, D. F. McCoy, and M. T. Bardo. 1990. "Conditioning of Morphine-Induced Taste Aversion and Analgesia." *Psychopharmacology,* 101:472–480.

Miller, N. E. 1969. "Learning of Visceral and Glandular Responses." *Science,* 163:434–445.

Miller, N. E., and B. Dworkin. 1980. "Different Ways in Which Learning Is Involved in Homeostasis. *Neural Mechanisms of Goal-Directed Behavior and Learning.* New York: Academic Press.

Moertel, C. G., W. F. Taylor, A. Roth, and F. A. J. Tyce. 1976. "Who Responds to Sugar Pills?" *Mayo Clinic Proceedings,* 51:96–100.

Moscucci, M., L. Byrne, M. Weintraub, and C. Cox. 1987. "Blinding, Unblinding, and the Placebo Effect: An Analysis of Patients' Guesses of Treatment Assignment in a Double-Blind Clinical Trial." *Clinical Pharmacology and Therapeutics,* 41:259–265.

Moynihan, J., D. Koota, G. Brenner, N. Cohen, and R. Ader. 1989. "Repeated Intraperitoneal Injections of Saline Attenuate the Antibody Response to a Subsequent Intraperitoneal Injection of Antigen." *Brain, Behavior, and Immunity,* 3:90–96.

Ney, P. G., C. Collins, and C. Spensor. 1986. "Double Blind: Double Talk or Are There Ways To Do Better Research?" *Medical Hypotheses,* 21:119–126.

Numan, R., N. Smith, and H. Lal. 1975. "Reduction of Morphine-Withdrawal Body Shakes by a Conditioned Stimulus in the Rat." *Psychopharmacology Communications,* 1:295–303.

Olness, K., and R. Ader. 1992. "Conditioning as an Adjunct in the Pharmacotherapy of Lupus Erythematosus: A Case Report." *Journal of Developmental and Behavioral Pediatrics,* 13:124–125.

Pavlov, I. P. 1927. *Conditioned Reflexes.* London: Oxford University Press.

Petrie, A. 1960. "Some Psychological Aspects of Pain and the Relief of Suffering." *Annals of the New York Academy of Science,* 86:13–27.

Pihl, R. O., and J. Altman. 1971. "An Experimental Analysis of the Placebo Effect." *Journal of Clinical Pharmacology,* 11:91–95.

Prien, R. F., J. O. Cole, and N. T. Belkin. 1968. "Relapse in Chronic Schizophrenics Following Abrupt Withdrawal of Tranquilizing Medication." *British Journal of Psychiatry,* 115:679–686.

Rickels, K., R. Lipmasn, and E. Raab. 1966. "Previous Medication, Duration of Illness and Placebo Response." *Journal of Nervous and Mental Disease,* 142:548–554.

Roffman, M., C. Reddy, and H. Lal. 1973. "Control of Morphine-Withdrawal Hypothermia by Conditioned Stimuli." *Psychopharmacologia,* 29:197–201.

Ross, S., and S. B. Schnitzer. 1963. "Further Support for the Placebo Effect in the Rat." *Psychological Reports,* 13:461–462.

Rozin, P., and J. W. Kalat. 1971. "Specific Hungers and Poison Avoidance as Adaptive Specializations of Learning." *Psychological Review,* 78:459–486.

Shaskin, E. G., and E. J. Lovett, III. 1981. "Effects of Haloperidol, a Dopamine Receptor Antagonist, on a Delayed-Type Hypersensitivity Reaction to 1-Chloro-2–4-Dinitrobenzene in Mice." *Research Communications in Psychology, Psychiatry, and Biology,* 5:241–254.

Sherman, J. E. 1979. "The Effects of Conditioning and Novelty on the Rat's Analgesic and Pyretic Responses to Morphine." *Learning and Motivation,* 10:383–418.

Siegel, S. 1983. "Classical Conditioning, Drug Tolerance, and Drug Dependence." *Research Advances in Alcohol and Drug Problems,* 7:207–246.

Skinner, B. F. 1953. *Science and Human Behavior.* London: MacMillan.

Stanley, W. C., and H. Schlosberg. 1953. "The Psychophysiological Effects of Tea." *Journal of Psychology,* 36:435–448.

Storlien, L. H., and D. J. Smith, D. M. Atrens, and P. F. Loribund. 1985. "Development of Hypoglycemia and Hyperglycemia as a Function of Number of Trials in Insulin Conditioning." *Physiology and Behavior,* 35:603–606.

Suchman, A., and R. Ader. 1992. "Classic Conditioning and Placebo Effects in Crossover Studies." *Clinical Pharmacology and Therapeutics,* 52:372–377.

Sunshine, A., E. Laska, M. Meisner, and S. Morgan. 1964. "Analgesic Studies of Indomethacin as Analyzed by Computer Techniques." *Clinical Pharmacology and Therapeutics,* 5:699–707.

Thomson, R. 1982. "Side Effects in Placebo Amplification." *British Journal of Psychiatry,* 140:64–68.

Voudouris, N. J., C. L. Peck, and G. Coleman. 1985. "Conditioned Placebo Responses." *Journal of Personality and Social Psychology,* 48:453–457.

White, L., B. Tursky, and G. Schwartz, eds. 1985. *Placebo: Theory, Research, and Mechanisms.* New York: Guilford Press.

Wickramasekera, I. 1980. "A Conditioned Response Model of the Placebo Effect: Predictions From the Model." *Biofeedback and Self Regulation,* 5:5–18.

Wikler, A. 1973. "Dynamics of Drug Dependence: Implications of a Conditioning Theory for Research and Treatment." *Archives of General Psychiatry,* 28:611–616.

Wolf, S. 1950. "Effects of Suggestion and Conditioning on the Action of Chemical Agents in Human Subjects—The Pharmacology of Placebos." *Journal of Clinical Investigation,* 29:100–109.

Zwyghuizen-Doorenbos, A., T. A. Roehrs, L. Lipschutz, V. Timms, and T. Roth. 1990. *Psychopharmacology,* 100:36–39.

Acknowledgments

Preparation of this chapter was supported by a Research Scientist Award (KO5 MH06318) and a Research Grant (MH42051) from the National Institute of Mental Health.

Specifying Nonspecifics: Psychological Mechanisms of Placebo Effects

8

Irving Kirsch

The placebo effect paradigm is as follows: a patient or research participant is given an inert substance and led to believe that it has physical properties that produce particular effects. He or she reports experiencing the expected effects. Because the treatment does not in fact have the physical properties ascribed to it, it is generally assumed that the effects are due to the recipients' beliefs and expectations.

I have labeled the beliefs that appear to mediate placebo effects *response expectancies* (Kirsch 1985, 1990). Response expectancies are anticipations of the occurrence of nonvolitional responses, such as pain, sadness, joy, intoxication, vomiting, and alertness. They can be distinguished from *stimulus expectancies,* which are anticipations of the occurrence of external consequences, such as food, money, praise, and punishment. Response expectancies can also be distinguished from anticipations of voluntary responses, which have been labeled *intentions* in the psychological literature (Ajzen and Fishbein 1980). The phenomena of placebo effects suggest that response expectancies are self-confirming.

Although the idea that placebo effects are mediated by expectancy may seem self-evident, at least two alternate explanations have been proposed. One explanation is that the effects are not real; the other is that they are due to classical conditioning and that the expectancies they elicit are epiphenomenal. This chapter provides a review of the data pertinent to these three competing hypotheses.

166

Placebo Effects as Artifacts

Some explanations of placebo effects imply that the effects are more apparent than real. These include the hypotheses that placebo effects are due to spontaneous remission, compliance with demand, or perceptual bias. This section reviews the data indicating that placebos can produce genuine effects that cannot be so easily dismissed.

Spontaneous Remission

Although some apparent placebo effects may be due to spontaneous remission, others clearly are not. Meta-analysis indicates a change of 1.12 standard deviations on measures of depression following administration of placebo antidepressants, compared with a change of 0.35 standard deviations among untreated controls and 1.54 standard deviations following administration of active drugs (Sapirstein 1995). These data indicate that 23 percent of the response to antidepressant medication is due to spontaneous remission, 27 percent is due to the drug, and 50 percent is due to expectancy. Similarly, placebo analgesics, tranquilizers, stimulants, and alcohol have been found to produce effects beyond those observed in untreated control conditions (Abrams and Wilson 1979; Baker and Kirsch 1993; Blackwell, Bloomfield, and Buncher 1972; Briddell et al. 1978; Brodeur 1965; Buckalew 1972; Camatte, Gerolami, and Searles 1969; Fillmore, Mulvihill, and Vogel-Sprott 1994; Fillmore and Vogel-Sprott 1992; Frankenhaeuser et al. 1963; Frankenhaeuser et al. 1964; Gelfand, Ullmann, and Krasner 1963; Kirsch and Weixel 1988; Lang et al. 1975; Lang et al. 1980; Lansky and Wilson 1981; Liberman 1964; Lyerly et al. 1964; Montgomery and Kirsch, in press; Morris and O'Neal 1974; Ross et al. 1962; Wilson and Abrams 1977; Wilson and Lawson 1976).

Compliance with Demand and Perceptual Bias

Experimental subjects are often able to divine the experimental hypotheses and may be motivated to please the experimenter by confirming it (Orne 1969). Similarly, patients may be motivated to confirm the expectations of healers. Alternately, the expectation of a change in experience may produce a perceptual bias, so that patients or research participants mistakenly perceive a change that has not in fact occurred.

Because many of the established effects of placebos are based on self-reported experience, the possibility of deception and self-deception cannot be ruled out. Conversely, deception and self-deception are unlikely explanations for placebo effects on physiological conditions that are not under voluntary control. Unfortunately, many of the reports purporting to demonstrate effects of this sort are anecdotal or uncontrolled. The well-known case report of an exceptionally powerful placebo effect on a malignant tumor (Klopfer 1957) has never been followed up with controlled research. Placebo-induced changes in gastric acid secretion and gastric contractions were described by Wolf and his colleagues (Abbot, Mack, and Wolf 1952; Wolf 1950), but the only controlled study of the effects of placebo on gastric function failed to find significant effects (Tyler 1946). Although reported placebo effects on warts in uncontrolled studies exceeded spontaneous remission rates obtained from other studies (Allington 1952), the results of controlled comparisons have been equivocal (Memmesheimer and Eisenlohr 1931; Spanos, Stenstrom, and Johnston 1988; Spanos, Williams, and Gwynn 1990).

In contrast to these anecdotal and uncontrolled data, Ikemi and Nakagawa (1962) reported a nicely designed within-subject study of suggestion-related production and inhibition of contact dermatitis. Thirteen hypersensitive subjects were touched on one arm with leaves from a harmless tree but were told that the leaves were from a lacquer or wax tree (Japanese trees that produce effects similar to poison ivy). On the other arm, the subjects were touched with irritant leaves, which they were led to believe were from a harmless tree. All thirteen subjects displayed a skin reaction to the harmless leaves (the placebo), but only two reacted to the irritant leaves. The dramatic nature of these results leaves one wishing for an independent replication.

Deception and self-deception can also be ruled out when self-reports of subjective change are accompanied by corresponding physiological changes. The inhibition of placebo analgesic effects by the injection of naloxone supports the validity of self-reported pain reduction (Fields and Levine 1981), and controlled studies indicate that placebos can induce and at least partially reverse bronchoconstriction in asthmatics

(Butler and Steptoe 1986; Godfrey and Silverman 1973; Horton et al. 1978; Luparello et al. 1968; Spector et al. 1976; Strupp et al. 1974). Similarly, self-reported arousal following placebo stimulants and tranquilizers has been accompanied by significant changes in heart rate and blood pressure (Frankenhaeuser et al. 1963; Kirsch and Weixel 1988); also, the effect of placebo alcohol on male sexual arousal has been supported by changes in heart rate, skin temperature, and penile tumescence (Briddell et al. 1978; Lang et al. 1980; Lansky and Wilson 1981; Wilson and Lawson 1976). These data convincingly demonstrate that many self-reported placebo effects reflect an actual change in condition.

Classical Conditioning

There are at least three ways of understanding classical conditioning: the traditional stimulus substitution model, the reinterpreted stimulus substitution model, and the cognitive or informational model. This section describes both stimulus substitution models and reviews data specific to each. Because the cognitive model is consistent with expectancy theory, it is described and evaluated in a subsequent section.

The Traditional Stimulus Substitution Model

According to the traditional stimulus substitution model, conditioning occurs when an initially neutral stimulus, called the *conditional stimulus (CS),* is paired with an *unconditional stimulus (US),* which is a stimulus that reliably elicits a particular response, called the *unconditional response (UR).* As a result of repeated pairing of the CS with the US, the CS comes to elicit the response even when presented alone. When elicited by the CS, the response is termed a *conditional response (CR).* This model of classical conditioning eliminates the need for cognitive or mentalistic concepts in explanations of learning.

Pavlovian explanations of placebo effects have been based on this traditional model of classical conditioning (Ader and Cohen 1991; Herrnstein 1962; Wickramasekera 1980). Active ingredients are USs, and the vehicles in which they are delivered (i.e., the pills, capsules, syringes, and so on) are CSs. The medical treatments that people experience during their lives constitute conditioning trials, during which the vehicles are paired with their active ingredients. These pairings endow the pills, capsules, and injections with the capacity to evoke therapeutic effects as CRs. Support for the traditional stimulus substitution model of placebo effects has been drawn from reports of the use of drugs as USs in conditioning experiments with laboratory animals (Herrnstein 1962; Pavlov 1927; Ross and Schnitzer 1963) and human subjects (Suchman and Ader 1992; Zwyghuizen-Doorenbos et al. 1990). Data demonstrating conditioned immunosuppression also support a stimulus substitution model of placebo effects (Ader and Cohen 1991).

In contrast to these data, conditioning with various drugs as USs has been reported to result in CRs that are the opposite of the URs (Siegel 1983), a finding that is inconsistent with the traditional stimulus substitution model. For example, whereas the US to morphine is a decrease in pain sensitivity, the CR to a stimulus that has been paired with morphine is an increase in pain sensitivity. Similarly, although tranquilizers like chlorpromazine reduce activity levels, the CR to stimuli with which they have been paired is to increase activity levels in laboratory animals. These data are especially important because the effects of placebo analgesics and tranquilizers are particularly well established.

The Revised Stimulus Substitution Model

Eikelboom and Stewart (1982) have proposed a reinterpretation of the stimulus substitution model, aimed at accounting for the apparently paradoxical phenomenon of CRs that are in the opposite direction of the URs. According to their model, active drugs are USs only if they affect the afferent or input arm of the central nervous system, and their effects are URs only if they are centrally mediated. These are the instances in which the CR should be the same as the UR. In contrast, if the drug affects the efferent arm of the nervous system without central mediation, the drug response is the US rather than the UR, and the CR will be a response that opposes or counteracts the drug effect.

The problem with this model, as it applies to placebo effects, is that it predicts the opposite response of that typically observed when humans ingest placebos. Recall that in conditioning studies, a CS paired with morphine produces hyperalgesia as a CR, and a CS paired with a tranquilizer (chlorpromazime) produces increased activity (Siegel 1983). In contrast, placebo morphine reduces pain, and placebo tranquilizers decrease activity levels in human subjects (Evans 1974; Frankenhaeuser et al. 1963, 1964). Consistent with Eikelboom and Stewart's (1982) interpretation of stimulus substitution, the administration of active medication to pain patients weakens subsequent placebo responses (Batterman and Lower 1968), as does the administration of active tranquilizers to psychiatric patients (Meath et al. 1956; Rickels, Lipman, and Raab 1966; Segal and Shapiro 1959; Zukin, Arnold, and Kessler 1959). These data indicate that conditioning with analgesics and tranquilizers produce compensatory responses. But if the CR to these drugs is a compensatory response, then the positive placebo responses that are partially reversed by conditioning occur in spite of—rather than because of—classical conditioning. Instead of explaining placebo effects, these data indicate that placebo-induced expectancies are able to reverse the effects of classical conditioning.

Expectancy Theory

The Eikelboom and Stewart (1982) model is an elaboration of the traditional stimulus substitution model of Pavlovian conditioning. However, research in the broader field of classical conditioning over the past thirty years has led to the replacement of stimulus substitution models by a conception of conditioning phenomena that is consistent with expectancy theory (Rescorla 1988). An example of the kind of data leading to the rejection of stimulus substitution models is the finding that under certain circumstances, the pairing of a CS with a US does not lead to associative learning. The common feature of these circumstances is the fact that the information value of the CS as a predictor of the US is blocked or masked. For example, if the US has a high base rate of occurrence in the absence of the CS, the effect of US–CS pairings can be negligible. Data of this sort have led contemporary theorists to describe conditioning as the learning of relations between events. Conditioning leads to the acquisition of expectancies that certain events will follow other events, and its occurrence depends on "the information that the CS provides about the US" (Rescorla 1988, p. 153), rather than on contiguity. The UR can be viewed as an anticipatory response that prepares the organism for the occurrence of the anticipated US (Siegel 1983). The response may be compensatory (for example, when performance inhibition is anticipated) or preparatory (for example, when food is anticipated).

The application of a contemporary informational view of classical conditioning to placebo phenomena (Kirsch 1990) shares some similarities with the Eikelboom and Stewart (1982) stimulus substitution model. It begins with the premise that for a stimulus to function as a US, it has to be perceived. But the active nature of a drug with which its vehicle is paired is perceived only by its effects. Therefore, in terms of information value, the drug response is the US, rather than the UR. What is learned during conditioning is that alcohol produces intoxication, stimulants increase arousal, analgesics reduce pain, and so on. Thus, classical conditioning is a means by which the response expectancies that mediate placebo effects are acquired (Kirsch 1990). However, conditioning is not the only means by which expectancies are formed. We also acquire them through reading, listening, and observing the behavior of others. The effect of placebos depends on the strength of the person's expectancies, not on how those expectations were formed.

Strong support for the response expectancy model of placebo effects is provided by data indicating that the response to placebo analgesics and tranquilizers is the opposite of the CR to the active drugs (see the data reviewed in the previous section). Thus, when conditioning produces effects that are contrary to people's expectancies, the effect of expectancy may be powerful enough to reverse the conditioning effect. Additional support for the expectancy model can be drawn from data demonstrating placebo responses that are unrelated to actual drug effects, from studies in which conditioning was blocked by providing verbal information, and from failures of placebo responses to extinguish despite repeated unreinforced administrations. These data are reviewed in the following sections.

Unconditioned Placebo Effects

According to stimulus substitution models, the placebo should affect the same responses that are affected by the active drug (although the direction of the response may vary as a function of the site of drug action). This does not seem to be the case with respect to placebo alcohol. Placebo alcohol produces a wide variety of effects that are orthogonal to the pharmacological effects of alcohol. That is, responses produced by alcohol (for example, cognitive-motor deficits) are not produced by placebo alcohol, and responses elicited by placebo alcohol (for example, increased craving) are not produced by surreptitiously administered alcohol (Hull and Bond 1986). Instead of being specific to the pharmacological properties of alcohol, the effects of placebo alcohol are specific to beliefs that vary from one culture to another (MacAndrew and Edgerton 1969). Similarly, the effects of placebo caffeine on motor performance vary as a function of the person's beliefs (Fillmore et al. 1994; Fillmore and Vogel-Sprott 1992; Kirsch and Weixel 1988). The placebo caffeine effects impede motor performance in people who expect that effect and enhance performance in people holding positive expectancies.

The Effect of Verbal Information on Conditioning Procedures

Apparent support for a classical conditioning model of placebo analgesia was reported by Voudouris, Peck, and Coleman (1985), who found an enhanced placebo effect following a series of conditioning trials during which the intensity of a pain stimulus was surreptitiously lowered when paired with placebo administration. In a subsequent study, they showed that this conditioning effect was greater than that of a verbal expectancy manipulation (Voudouris et al. 1990). From a cognitive perspective, however, conditioning trials are themselves expectancy manipulations. So what was demonstrated by Voudouris et al. (1990) can be interpreted as indicating that experiential manipulations (that is, conditioning trials) are more effective than verbal manipulations in altering expectancies, a finding that had previously been reported by expectancy theorists (Wickless and Kirsch 1989).

Montgomery and Kirsch (in press) conducted an empirical comparison of stimulus substitution and response expectancy interpretations of conditioned placebo effects. In addition to replicating the conditioning procedure used by Voudouris et al. (1985, 1990), Montgomery included an informed pairing conditioning group and an extinction control group. The informed pairing condition differed from the usual conditioning group in that subjects were told that the stimulus intensity was being lowered during conditioning trails. If the conditioning effect is a direct consequence of CS–US pairings, it should not be blocked by informing subjects of the manipulation. Conversely, if the conditioning effect is mediated by expectancy, nondeceptive pairings should fail to produce conditioning. Consistent with the expectancy interpretation, an increase in the placebo effect was obtained only when subjects were deceived into thinking that the intensity of the pain stimulus had been held constant. Furthermore, changes in pain reduction were accompanied by corresponding changes in expected pain reduction, indicating that the effect of the conditioning trials was mediated by expectancy.

Resistance to Extinction

According to classical conditioning theories, repeated presentation of the CS alone should result in extinction of the CR. Contrary to this prediction, placebo effects can be very long lasting. In the experimental study of conditioned analgesia described in the previous section, Montgomery and Kirsch (in press) found that the magnitude of the effect of placebo analgesia increased, rather than decreased, across ten extinction trials. In clinical studies, eight weeks of daily placebo administration failed to reduce the effectiveness of placebo treatment for panic disorder (Coryell and Noyes 1988); placebos retained their effectiveness in the treatment of angina over a six-month period (Boissel et al. 1986); and continued placebo treatment of rheumatoid arthritis was shown to be effective for as long as thirty months (Traut and Passarelli 1957). These examples could hardly be described as extinction curves!

Although it is difficult to reconcile these data with a stimulus substitution model of conditioning, they are not inconsistent with an expectancy interpretation. According to the response expectancy hypothesis, response expectancies are self-confirming. Therefore, once the expectancy has been produced, there is no need for further reinforcement by a US. Instead, the response produced by the expectancy confirms the expectancy. Extinction of the placebo response requires disconfirmation of the placebo-induced expectancy. For example, one might lead a person to conclude that the placebo had lost its potency by surreptitiously increasing the intensity of the pain stimulus, as shown by Voudouris et al. (1985).

Taken as a whole, the data strongly disconfirm the classical conditioning model of placebo effects. Conditioning seems to have at least two types of effects. One of these occurs through stimulus substitution and is not mediated by expectancy. But many of the conditional responses established through stimulus substitution are compensatory in nature. Their effect is to inhibit, rather than to produce, the placebo effect. Thus, the effects of expectancy appear to be stronger than the effects of stimulus substitution.

Conditioning trials also produce expectancies, but this effect is not automatic; instead, it depends on the information that is available to the person. Furthermore, conditioning is not the only means by which expectancies are acquired. Expectancies can also be acquired vicariously, as seems to be the case with some widely held, but erroneous, beliefs about the effect of alcohol. Most importantly, the effects of placebo alcohol indicate that when what is expected is different from the response to the US, the observed response is the one that the person expects. What remains to be explained, however, is how response expectancies produce the expected response. This question is addressed in the following section.

How Do Expectancies Affect Responses?

Among the variables hypothesized to mediate the relation between expectancy and placebo response are trust, faith, hopefulness, anxiety reduction, endorphin release, and the therapeutic relationship. Although all of these factors may be involved in some instances of placebo responding, this section demonstrates that none of the factors can account for the full range of placebo effects. The consistency of the placebo effect (that is, the fact that it almost always corresponds to the recipient's beliefs about the active drug), combined with the continuing failure to find a mediating variable that can account for the available data, leads me to suggest that some of the effects of expectancy may be direct, rather than mediated.

The Therapeutic Relationship

Among the most well-established effects of placebos are those of placebo analgesics, tranquilizers, stimulants, and alcohol (see citations in the sections on spontaneous remission). The authenticity of these effects has been verified by comparison with untreated controls and by the observation of concomitant changes in physiological function. These changes could not have been due to the therapeutic relationship, because most of these studies were conducted on healthy volunteers in relatively sterile, nonclinical, experimental settings. Nor is hopefulness likely to be a factor. Not only were the research participants in these studies not ill, but also there is no reason to presume that they felt hopeless when they volunteered for the studies. Nor is there any reason to suppose that the thought of getting a tranquilizer or stimulant would make them feel hopeful about anything.

Even in clinical situations, the effects of placebos cannot be due entirely to the therapeutic relationship. For example, placebo injections are more effective than placebo pills in reducing clinical pain (Traut and Passarelli 1957). Because the relationship was the same in both conditions, it could not have been responsible for the observed differences in the placebo response.

The Specificity of Placebo Effects

The popular definition of *placebo* as "nonspecific" treatment is not entirely accurate. Although the ingredients of a placebo preparation may be unspecific, the effects of placebos are very specific, and an adequate explanation of placebo effects must account for that specificity.

The specific nature of the effects of placebos (that is, whether the placebo affects gastric motility, sexual arousal, pain perception, and so on) depends on the information available to the recipient. For example, placebos given as tranquilizers produce very different effects from the same placebos presented as stimulants (Frankenhaeuser et al. 1963). Similarly, the side effects produced by placebos vary as a function of the recipient's knowledge about the active drug. Vomiting, for example, is reported as a side effect by approximately 8 percent of subjects given placebo estrogen, but by less than 0.01 percent of subjects given placebos for other substances (Pogge 1963). It is difficult to imagine how such "nonspecific" factors as hope and faith could produce such specific effects.

The unwanted side effects produced by placebos present a particular problem for the hypothesis that placebo effects are due to hope and optimism. Frank (1973) has explained the occurrence of these effects as being due to fear of drugs and distrust of doctors. However, positive and negative effects frequently occur in the same person and are sometimes positively correlated (Loranger, Prout, and White 1961; Rickels et al. 1967; Shapiro, Struening, and Shapiro 1980). These data cannot be explained by such hypotheses as faith, trust, hopefulness, or the therapeutic relationship. A person does not feel hopeful and hopeless or trusting and untrusting at the same time.

Finally, data from my laboratory (Montgomery and Kirsch 1996) indicate that at least some types of placebo pain reduction cannot be explained by mechanisms that would affect the entire body (for instance, anxiety reduction or endorphin release). We obtained a placebo effect by administering the placebo in the guise of a local anesthetic and applying a pain stimulus to treated and untreated parts of the body. Because the pain stimulus was applied simultaneously to both the treated (by placebo) and untreated locations, the differences in reported pain could not have been due to any global changes in sensitivity, perception, or affect.

How can our data be reconciled with those indicating that naloxone, an opioid antagonist, can block the effect of placebo analgesia? The effects of placebos generally mimic the effects of the active drugs bearing their label. Therefore, the effects of placebos presented as general analgesics might be different from those of placebos presented as topical anesthetics. Placebo opiates engender expectancies of the altered state of consciousness produced by actual opiates. Those expectancies may produce some features of those altered states, and in so doing, they may be accompanied by the release of endogenous opioids in the brain. In contrast, people receiving what they believe to be a topical anesthetic would not anticipate an altered state of consciousness. Thus, both types of placebo should reduce pain, but pain reduction should be associated with endorphin release only when the placebo is presented as a general analgesic.

Unmediated Expectancy Effects

The question "How does the expectancy of a change in subjective experience produce that change?" generates a search for mediating variables. However, there must be at least some relations between causal and consequential psychological variables that are not psychologically mediated, or else there would be an infinite regress. At some point, the search for psychological mediators must come to an end. At that point, further elaboration of explanatory mechanisms requires consideration of the physiological substrates of psychological variables.

Ajzen and Fishbein (1980) use the term *immediate* to describe the relation between two variables that are causally related with no intervening variable mediating the relation. They use this term not in the conventional sense but as an antonym for *mediated*. Their example of an immediate relation is that between an intention and an intended volitional act. The claim is that there are no intervening psychological variables between the intention and the intended response.

Other examples of immediate relations between cognitions and psychological responses are those between perceived threat and fear and between perceived loss and sadness. Fear is an immediate consequence of the expectation of an aversive or harmful event, and sadness is an immediate consequence of the belief that one has irretrievably lost something of great consequence (Beck 1976). Similarly, I have suggested that the occurrence of a subjective experience may be an immediate consequence of its expectation (Kirsch 1985, 1990).

In some instances, the immediacy of the connection between a response expectancy and the subjective experience that it affects is intuitively obvious. For example, many people find the experience of fear extremely aversive. Because the experience of fear is so aversive for these individuals, the anticipation of its occurrence is a fear-inducing cognition. This is why the panic experienced by agoraphobics is so often described as a "fear of fear." Agoraphobics do not fear the supermarkets, shopping malls, elevators, bridges, automobiles, or open spaces that they avoid. Instead, they fear the panic attack that they expect to experience in those places. When they are unable to avoid the situations in which they expect to panic, their expectancy of this highly aversive outcome produces fear of fear, which recursively escalates into a full-blown panic attack (Goldstein and Chambless 1978). There are ample data indicating that expected fear is an important causal factor, not only in agoraphobia but also in other phobic disorders as well (Gauthier et al. 1987; Kirsch and Henry 1977; Kirsch et al. 1983; Southworth and Kirsch 1988).

The phenomenology of depression provides another intuitively clear link between expectancy and subjective response. For many depressed individuals, the experience of depression is the most depressing aspect of their lives. These individuals have been described as depressed about their own depression (Teasdale 1985). They expect to remain depressed, and because depression is aversive, the expectation that it will persist is an extremely depressing thought. The administration of a placebo elicits the belief that the depression will subside. To the extent that the depression was maintained by the expectancy that it would not abate, the placebo may be sufficient to relieve it.

The reason for an immediate link between expectancy and expected response is not always clear. For example, it is not clear why the expectation of nausea in chemotherapy patients produces anticipatory nausea; why a verbally induced expectancy for mirth produces that feeling (Wilson et al. 1989); or why expectancies of pain, relaxation, alertness, and sexual arousal produce those feelings. Nevertheless, the consistency of the relation between response expectancies and subsequent responses suggests of a general mechanism linking the expectancy of subjective reactions to their occurrence, and the failure to find a mediating variable capable of accounting for all of these effects suggests that the relation may be immediate.

Physiological Effects of Placebos

I have proposed the immediacy hypothesis only for subjective effects of response expectancies. However, placebos have also been shown to affect physiological functions. These effects are of two types. There are well-established effects on responses that are part of the physiological substrate of subjective experiences. Examples of this type of placebo effect include the effect of placebo tranquilizers and stimulants on heart rate and blood pressure and the effect of placebo alcohol on penile tumescence. The specificity of these effects suggest that the search for physiological mechanisms will require discovering the physiological substrates of specific expectations, such as the expectancy that the left index finger, but not other parts of the body, will be less sensitive to pain (Montgomery and Kirsch 1996).

Placebos have also been reported to affect physiological responses that are not part of the physiological substrates of subjective experience. The effect of placebos on skin conditions (warts and contact dermatitis), cancer, and the immune function are examples of this second type of physiological placebo effect. Some of the reported effects of this sort seem amazing (Ikemi and Nakagawa 1962; Klopfer 1957), and if substantiated, they are exceptionally important. Unfortunately, the data for this type of placebo effect are either equivocal, anecdotal, or unreplicated. Therefore, the first order of business is to establish their reliability and magnitude.

If these effects can be verified, a search for mediating psychological mechanisms will be justified. Unlike placebo effects on subjective reactions and their substrates, data have not yet established the specificity of the hypothesized effects of placebos on physiological functions that are not substrates of psychological states. The questions is this: are these effects specific to the activation of particular response expectancies, as seems to be the case with the effects of placebo tranquilizers, stimulants, and alcohol, or are they a function of more global psychological changes, such as changes in anxiety, hopefulness, and depression?

Conclusion

A review of the experimental data indicates that many placebo effects are genuine and should not be regarded merely as artifacts. These effects cannot be explained by classical conditioning. With some drugs, conditioning procedures produce conditioned responses that are directly opposite of placebo responses. In these cases, placebo effects occur in spite of conditioning, rather than because of it. In other cases, conditioning may be a means by which placebo expectancies are produced, but it is the expectancy, rather than the pairing of conditional and unconditional stimuli, that produces the placebo response. Placebo effects illustrate a basic principle of psychological functioning: the self-confirming nature of response expectancy.

References

Abbot, F. K., M. Mack, and S. Wolf. 1952. "The Action of Banthine on the Stomach and Duodenum of Man with Observations of the Effects of Placebos." *Gastroenterology*, 20:249–269.

Abrams, D. B., and G. T. Wilson. 1979. "Effects of Alcohol on Anxiety in Women: Cognitive Versus Physiological Processes." *Journal of Abnormal Psychology,* 88:161–173.

Ader, R., and N. Cohen. 1991. "The Influence of Conditioning on Immune Responses." In R. Ader, D. L. Felten, and N. Cohen, eds., *Psychoneuro-immunology,* 2nd ed. San Diego: Academic Press, p. 611–646.

Ajzen, I., and M. Fishbein. 1980. *Understanding Attitudes and Predicting Social Behavior.* Englewood Cliffs, N.J.: Prentice-Hall.

Allington, H. V. 1952. "Review of the Psychotherapy of Warts." *A.M.A. Archives of Dermatology and Syphilology,* 66:316–326.

Baker, S. L., and I. Kirsch. 1993. "Hypnotic and Placebo Analgesia: Order Effects and the Placebo Label." *Contemporary Hypnosis,* 10:117–126.

Batterman, R. C., and W. R. Lower. 1968. "Placebo-responsiveness—The Influence of Previous Therapy." *Current Therapeutic Research,* 10:136–143.

Beck, A. T. 1976. *Cognitive Therapy and the Emotional Disorders.* New York: International Universities Press.

Blackwell, B., S. S. Bloomfield, and C. R. Buncher. 1972. "Demonstration to Medical Students of Placebo Responses and Non-drug Factors." *The Lancet,* 19:1279–1282.

Boissel, J. P., A. M. Philippon, E. Gauthier, J. Schbath, J. M. Destors, and the B.I.S. Research Group. 1986. "Time Course of Long-term Placebo Therapy Effects in Angina Pectoris." *European Heart Journal,* 7:1030–1036.

Briddell, D. W., D. C. Rimm, G. W. Caddy, G. Krawitz, D. Sholis, and R. J. Wunderlin. 1978. "The Effects of Alcohol and Cognitive Set on Sexual Arousal to Deviant Stimuli." *Journal of Abnormal Psychology,* 87:418–430.

Brodeur, D. W. 1965. "The Effects of Stimulant and Tranquilizer Placebos on Healthy Subjects in a Real-life Situation." *Psychopharmacologia,* 7:444–452.

Buckalew, L. W. 1972. "An Analysis of Experimental Components in a Placebo Effect." *The Psychological Record,* 22:113–119.

Butler, C., and A. Steptoe. 1986. "Placebo Responses: An Experimental Study of Psychophysiological Processes in Asthmatic Volunteers." *British Journal of Clinical Psychology,* 25:173–183.

Camatte, R., A. Gerolami, and H. Sarles. 1969. "Comparative Study of the Action of Different Treatments and Placebos on Pain Crises of Gastro-duodenal Ulcers." *Clinica Terapeutica,* 49:411–419.

Coryell, W., and R. Noyes. 1988. "Placebo Response in Panic Disorder." *American Journal of Psychiatry,* 145:1138–1140.

Eikelboom, R., and J. Stewart. 1982. "Conditioning of Drug-induced Physiological Responses." *Psychological Review,* 89:507–528.

Evans, F. J. 1974. "The Placebo Response in Pain Reduction." *Advances in Neurology,* 4:289–296.

Fields, H. L., and J. D. Levine. 1981. "Biology of Placebo Analgesia." *American Journal of Medicine,* 70:745–746.

Fillmore, M., L. E. Mulvihill, and M. Vogel-Sprott. 1994. "The Expected Drug and Its Expected Effect Interact to Determine Placebo Responses to Alcohol and Caffeine." *Psychopharmacology,* 115:383–388.

Fillmore, M., and M. Vogel-Sprott. 1992. "Expected Effect of Caffeine on Motor Performance Predicts the Type of Response to Placebo." *Psychopharmacology,* 106:209–214.

Frank, J. D. 1973. *Persuasion and Healing* (rev. ed.). Baltimore: Johns Hopkins.

Frankenhaeuser, M., G. Jarpe, H. Svan, and B. Wrangsjö. 1963. "Physiological Reactions to Two Different Placebo Treatments." *Scandinavian Journal of Psychology,* 4:245–250.

Frankenhaeuser, M., B. Post, R. Hagdahl, and B. Wrangsjö. 1964. "Effects of a Depressant Drug as Modified Experimentally-induced Expectation." *Perceptual and Motor Skills,* 18:513–522.

Gauthier, J. G., B. Laberge, L. Dufour, and A. Fevre. 1987. "Therapeutic Expectancies and Exposure in the Treatmaent of Phobic Anxiety." In S. L. Williams (Chair), Psychological Mechanisms in Performance Based Treatment of Severe Phobias. Symposium conducted at the meeting of the American Psychological Association, New York, August.

Gelfand, S., L. P. Ullmann, and L. Krasner. 1963. "The Placebo Response: An Experimental Approach." *Journal of Nervous and Mental Disease,* 136:379–387.

Godfrey, S., and M. Silverman. 1973. "Demonstration of the Placebo Response in Asthma by Means of Exercise Testing." *Journal of Psychosomatic Research,* 17:293–297.

Goldstein, A. J., and D. L. Chambless. 1978. "A Reanalysis of Agoraphobia." *Behavior Therapy,* 9:47–59.

Greenberg, R. P., and S. Fisher. 1989. "Examining Antidepressant Effectiveness: Findings, Ambiguities, and Some Vexing Puzzles." In S. Fisher and R. P. Greenberg, eds., *The Limits of Biological Treatments for Psychological Distress: Comparisons With Psychotherapy and Placebo.* Hillsdale, N.J.: Lawrence Erlbaum, p. 1–37.

Herrnstein, R. 1962. "Placebo Effect in the Rat." *Science,* 138:677–678.

Horton, D. J., W. L. Suda, R. A. Kinsman, J. Souhrada, and S. L. Spector. 1978. "Bronchoconstrictive Suggestion in Asthma: A Role for Airways Hyperreactivity and Emotions." *American Review of Respiratory Disease,* 117:1029–1038.

Hull, J. G., and C. F. Bond. 1986. "Social and Behavioral Consequences of Alcohol Consumption and Expectancy: A Meta-analysis." *Psychological Bulletin,* 99:347–360.

Ikemi, Y., and S. Nakagawa. 1962. "A Psychosomatic Study of Contagious Dermatitis." *Kyoshu Journal of Medical Science,* 13:335–350.

Kirsch, I. 1985. "Response Expectancy as a Determinant of Experience and Behavior." *American Psychologist,* 40:1189–1202.

———. 1990. *Changing Expectations: A Key to Effective Psychotherapy.* Pacific Grove, Calif: Brooks/Cole.

Kirsch, I., and D. Henry. 1977. "Extinction vs. Credibility in the Desensitization of Speech Anxiety." *Journal of Consulting and Clinical Psychology,* 45:1052–1059.

Kirsch, I., H. Tennen, C. Wickless, A. J. Saccone, and S. Cody. 1983. "The Role of Expectancy in Fear Reduction." *Behavior Therapy,* 14:520–533.

Kirsch, I., and L. J. Weixel. 1988. "Double-Blind Versus Deceptive Administration of a Placebo." *Behavioral Neuroscience,* 102:319–323.

Klopfer, B. 1957. "Psychological Variables in Human Cancer." *Journal of Projective Techniques,* 21:331–340.

Lang, A. R., D. J. Goeckner, V. J. Adesso, and G. A. Marlatt. 1975. "Effects of Alcohol on Aggression in Male Social Drinkers." *Journal of Abnormal Psychology,* 84:508–518.

Lang, A. R., J. Searles, R. Laurerman, and V. Adesso. 1980. "Expectancy, Alcohol, and Sex Guilt as Determinants of Interest in and Reaction to Sexual Stimuli." *Journal of Abnormal Psychology,* 89:644–653.

Lansky, D., and G. T. Wilson. 1981. "Alcohol, Expectations, and Sexual Arousal in Males: An Information Processing Analysis." *Journal of Abnormal Psychology,* 90:35–45.

Liberman, R. 1964. "An Experimental Study of the Placebo Response Under Three Different Situations of Pain." *Journal of Psychiatric Research,* 2:233–246.

Loranger, A. W., C. T. Prout, and M. A. White. 1961. "The Placebo Effect in Psychiatric Drug Research." *Journal of the American Medical Association,* 176:920–925.

Luparello, T. J., H. A. Lyons, E. R. Bleeker, E. R. McFadden. 1968. "Influence of Suggestion on Airways Reactivity in Asthmatic Subjects." *Psychosomatic Medicine,* 30:819.

Lyerly, S. B., S. Ross, A. D. Krugman, and D. J. Clyde. 1964. "Drugs and Placebos: The Effects of Instructions Upon Performance and Mood Under Amphetamine Sulphate and Chloral Hydrate." *Journal of Abnormal and Social Psychology,* 68:321–327.

MacAndrew, C., and R. B. Edgerton. 1969. *Drunken Comportment: A Social Explanation.* Chicago: Aldine-Atherton.

Meath, J. A., T. M. Feldberg, D. Rosenthal, and J. D. Frank. 1956. "Comparison of Reserpine and Placebo in Treatment of Psychiatric Outpatients." *A.M.A. Archives of Neurology and Psychiatry,* 76:207–214.

Memmesheimer, A. M., and E. Eisenlohr. 1931. "Untersuchungen über die suggestive behandlung der warzen." *Dermatol Zeitchr.,* 62:63–68.

Montgomery, G. H., and I. Kirsch. (in press). "Classical Conditioning and the Placebo Effect." *Pain.*

Montgomery, G., I. Kirsch. 1996. "Mechanisms of Placebo Pain Reduction: An Empirical Investigation." *Psychological Science,* 7:174–176.

Morris, L. A., and E. O'Neal. 1974. "Drug-name Familiarity and the Placebo Effect." *Journal of Clinical Psychology,* 30:280–282.

Orne, M. T. 1969. "Demand Characteristics and the Concept of Quasi-controls." In R. Rosenthal and R. L. Rosnow, eds. *Artifact in Behavioral Research.* New York: Academic Press, p. 143–179.

Pavlov, I. P. 1927. "Conditioned Reflexes." G. V. Anrep, Trans. New York: Liveright.

Pogge, R. 1963. "The Toxic Placebo." *Medical Times,* 91:773–778.

Rescorla, R. A. 1988. Pavlovian Conditioning: It's not what you think it is. *American Psychologist,* 43:151–160.

Rickels, K., Lipman, R., and Raab, E. 1966. "Previous Medication, Duration of Illness, and Placebo Response." *The Journal of Nervous and Mental Disease,* 142:548–554.

Rickels, K., L. Snow, H. Uhlenhuth, R. S. Lipman, L. C. Park, and S. Fisher. 1967. "Side Reactions on Meprobromate and Placebo." *Diseases of the Nervous System,* 28:39–45.

Ross, S., A. D. Krugman, S. B. Lyerly, and D. J. Clyde. 1962. "Drugs and Placebos: A Model Design." *Psychological Reports,* 10:383–392.

Ross, S., and S. B. Schnitzer. 1963. "Further Support for a Placebo Effect in the Rat." *Psychological Reports,* 13:461–462.

Sapirstein, G. 1995. "The Effectiveness of Placebos in the Treatment of Depression: A Meta-analysis." Unpublished doctoral dissertation, University of Connecticut, Storrs.

Segal, M., and K. L. Shapiro. 1959. "A Clinical Comparison Study of the Effects of Resperine and Placebo on Anxiety." *Archives of Neurology and Psychiatry,* 81:392–398.

Shapiro, A. K., E. Struening, and E. Shapiro. 1980. "The Reliability and Validity of a Placebo Test." *Journal of Psychiatric Research,* 15:253–290.

Siegel, S. 1983. "Classical Conditioning, Drug Tolerance, and Drug Dependence." In Y. Israel, F. B. Glaser, H. Kalant, R. E. Popham, W. Schmidt, and R. G. Smart, eds., *Research Advances in Alcohol and Drug Problems* (Vol. 7). New York: Plenum Press.

Southworth, S., and I. Kirsch. 1988. "The Role of Expectancy in Exposure-generated Fear Reduction in Agoraphobia." *Behaviour Research and Therapy,* 26:113–120.

Spanos, N. P., R. J. Stenstrom, and J. C. Johnston. 1988. "Hypnosis, Placebo, and Suggestion in the Treatment of Warts." *Psychosomatic Medicine,* 50:245–260.

Spanos, N. P., V. Williams, and M. I. Gwynn. 1990. "Effects of Hypnotic,

Placebo, and Salicylic Acid Treatments on Wart Regression." *Psychosomatic Medicine,* 52:109–114.

Spector, S. L., T. J. Luparello, M. T. Kopetzky, J. Souhrada, and R. A. Kinsman. 1976. "Response of Asthmatics to Methacholine and Suggestion." *American Review of Respiratory Disease,* 113:43–50.

Strupp, H. H., R. W. Levenson, S. B. Manuck, J. D. Snell, J. J. Hinrichsen, and S. Boyd. 1974. "Effects of Suggestion on Total Respiratory Resistance in Mild Asthmatics." *Journal of Psychosomatic Research,* 18:337–346.

Suchman, A. L., and R. Ader. 1992. "Classic Conditioning and Placebo Effects in Crossover Studies." *Clinical Pharmacology and Therapeutics,* 52:372–377.

Teasdale, J. D. 1985. "Psychological Treatments for Depression: How Do They Work?" *Behaviour Research and Therapy,* 23:157–165.

Traut, E. F., and E. W. Passarelli. 1957. "Placebos in the Treatment of Rheumatoid Arthritis and Other Rheumatic Conditions." *Annals of the Rheumatic Diseases,* 16:18–22.

Tyler, D. B. 1946. "The Influence of a Placebo, Body Position and Medication on Motion Sickness." *American Journal of Physiology,* 146:458–466.

Voudouris, N. J., C. L. Peck, and G. Coleman. 1985. "Conditioned Placebo Responses." *Journal of Personality and Social Psychology,* 48:47–53.

———. 1990. "The Role of Conditioning and Verbal Expectancy in the Placebo Response." *Pain,* 43:121–128.

Wickless, C., and I. Kirsch. 1989. "The Effects of Verbal and Experiential Expectancy Manipulations on Hypnotic Susceptibility." *Journal of Personality and Social Psychology,* 57:762–768.

Wickramasekera, I. 1980. "A Conditioned Response Model of the Placebo Effect: Predictions From the Model." *Biofeedback and Self-Regulation,* 5:5–18.

Wilson, G. T., and D. Abrams. 1977. "Effects of Alcohol on Social Anxiety and Physiological Arousal: Cognitive Versus Pharmacological Processes." *Cognitive Therapy and Research,* 1:195–210.

Wilson, G. T., and D. M. Lawson. 1976. "Expectancies, Alcohol, and Sexual Arousal in Male Social Drinkers." *Journal of Abnormal Psychology,* 85:587–594.

Wilson, T. D., D. J. Lisle, D. Kraft, and C. G. Wetzel. 1989. "Preferences as Expectation-driven Inferences: Effects of Affective Expectations on Affective Experience." *Journal of Personality and Social Psychology,* 56:519–530.

Wolf, S. 1950. "Effects of Suggestion and Conditioning on the Action of Chemical Agents in Human Subjects—The Pharmacology of Placebos." *Journal of Clinical Investigation,* 29:100–109.

Zukin, P., D. G. Arnold, and C. Kessler. 1959. "Comparative Effects of

Phenaglycodol and Meprobromate on Anxiety Reactions." *Journal of Nervous and Mental Disease,* 129:193–195.

Zwyghuizen-Doorenbos, A., R. A. Goehrs, L. Lipschutz, V. Timms, and T. Roth. 1990. "Effects of Caffeine on Alertness." *Psychopharmacology,* 100:36–39.

Placebo, Pain, and Belief: A Biocultural Model

9

David B. Morris

Placebo: an epithet given to any medicine adapted more
to please than to benefit the patient.

Hooper's Medical Dictionary (1811)

The term *placebo*—although employed in English since the time of Chaucer to denote sycophants or flatterers—enters the medical lexicon in 1811, bearing the still common implication that placebos are a kind of gratifying fraud, pleasant but useless. The date has a special significance. It binds placebos to the revolutionary moment in Western medicine that Michel Foucault (1973) has called the birth of the clinic. Among other changes, the ancient Galenic tradition that understood disease as an imbalance of internal forces and fluids—a disruption of the harmony linking microcosmic bodies with the divinely ordered macrocosm—was giving way to a clinically based experimental medicine rooted in a Cartesian dualism that redefined human bodies as machines. Split off equally from mind and from cosmos, a Cartesian body operates simply according to mechanical laws of matter and motion. Such mechanical laws, seemingly confirmed by nineteenth-century science through crucial discoveries about the nervous system, left no place for nonmedical cures or spontaneous relief. In the mechanistic tradition that still underlies much of modern biomedicine, believing in the power of a placebo to erase pain is as irrational as filling the gas tank of your car with Earl Grey tea.

Today, after nearly two hundred years banished to the limbo of quackery, placebos are starting to interest scientists and doctors. The interest is intermittent, regularly overwhelmed by irritation reserved for anomalies that complicate the mathematics of drug trials and defy rational explanation; but some researchers have finally come to review and to respect the evidence that placebos really work (Turner et al. 1994). Contrary to the widespread myth that one-third of all patients are placebo responders, the effectiveness of placebos ranges anywhere from 1 percent to 100 percent, depending on the conditions of the trial (Wall 1992). Indeed, placebos have proved effective in maladies that range all the way from depression and congestive heart failure to gastric ulcers and angina pectoris (Brown, Johnson, and Chen 1992; Archer and Leier 1992; Moerman 1983; Benson and McCallie 1979). It is true that placebos are not effective in some specific instances, such as intra-arterial ambulatory blood pressure and obsessive-compulsive disorder (Raftery and Gould 1990; Mavissakalian, Jones, and Olson 1990). Yet the demonstrable, if unexplained, therapeutic success of placebos means that the question today must be reframed not as whether placebos work but rather as *how* they work.

We still don't have a full answer, despite some attractive hypotheses, especially concerning the role of endorphins (Levine, Gordon, and Fields 1978). We don't even possess an inventory of exactly which medical conditions respond to placebos and how far the relief generated by placebos will extend. Can placebos shrink tumors? Stop asthma? Cure infections? Much detailed research is still needed. Researchers will continue to supply important details; however, we already know enough to discuss some fundamental issues. The fundamental claim that I wish to address here is the following: a full understanding of the placebo response in humans, like the phenomenon of pain with which it is so closely related, requires a biocultural model that acknowledges the intrinsic role of culture, meaning, and belief.

Physician Godehard Oepen, speaking at the 1994 Harvard University symposium on Placebo: Probing the Self-Healing Brain, put the basic fact about placebos quite clearly: "If you don't believe in them, they don't work." His statement—for which there is wide support (Wall 1993)—finds illustration in numerous colorful examples. In one study of ultrasound waves used to relieve pain following the extraction of wisdom teeth, patients got equally good pain relief no matter whether the ultrasound machine was turned on or off—so long as both patient and physician *believed* that it was turned on (Hashish et al. 1988). The placebo effect in this case extended not only to pain relief but also to a reduction of swelling. It is important to notice that physicians as well as patients contribute to the aura of belief. A British study (Thomas 1987) found that patients did appreciably less well than a control group if a physician told them "I am not sure what is the matter with you, and I am not sure the treatment will have an effect." Positive beliefs in the efficacy of medication or treatment are necessary to underwrite a placebo effect, while disbelief actively subverts it.

Placebos, in other words, place belief and meaning at the center of the therapeutic encounter. It thus requires something more than a neurobiological system to explain how placebos work in humans. Why, for example, do injections have a more potent placebo effect than pills, large pills a more potent effect than smaller pills, and very small pills a more potent effect than average-size pills? Research has shown that it is possible to create an apparent placebo response in lower animals simply by using the methods of classical conditioning (Voudouris, Peck, and Coleman 1989). Yet, while classic conditioning seems enough to evoke a placebo effect in rabbits and rats, and while humans too can be effectively conditioned to respond to a specific stimulus, such facts simply emphasize how important the cognitive dimension of placebos is in humans. These facts suggest that humans activate the neurobiological circuits required for placebo effects through the subtle and diffuse experience of living within the inescapably meaning-rich domain of culture.

The effectiveness of placebos shows up with great clarity in the case of pain. Analgesia is one of the most common and potent placebo effects. It seems, however, premature to say that *all* placebo effects employ the body's endogenous pain modulation systems with their reliance on spinal pathways and endorphin circuitry. Although researchers have not established the full range of medical conditions for which placebos are effective, it certainly extends far beyond pain. There is, however, one important way in which pain can serve as a useful paradigm of the placebo effect. No matter whether it is chronic or acute, pain depends on learning. The learning process begins in infancy, before we possess a language to assist and confuse us, and indeed requires no words at all. Pups isolated at birth in padded cells were later placed in a cage with low pipes overhead, where they were observed to bang their heads repeatedly, as if wholly unfamiliar with the experience of pain (Melzack 1960). Like other animals, humans first learn about pain by living in a material environment that confronts them with painful stimuli, while language and culture later provide still other complex systems through which our learning about pain is reinforced and extended. Indeed, the impact of language and culture is so powerful that it can completely reconstruct an individual's experience until (for some Christian mystics) pleasure is transformed into pain or (for Sade) pain is transformed into pleasure.

There is no doubt that culture communicates powerful and quite various lessons about pain. For example, the meanings and sources attributed to pain differ greatly across cultures and across time (Scarry 1985; Morris 1991). Tolerance for pain also varies widely not just among individuals but among groups. Prizefighters, Eskimos, day-laborers, Eastern mystics, and Romantic poets, that is, live a very different relation to pain than do stressed-out executives or victims of sexual abuse. Pain, then, offers an especially useful focus on the placebo effect because, despite the demonstrable role of nerves and neurotransmitters, it is always mediated by individual and cultural experience. Tissue damage alone does not correlate directly with pain, as is clear from studies of battlefield injuries. Soldiers in World War II tolerated terrible wounds without complaints of pain or requests for medication (Beecher 1946). Although a recent follow-up study based on the Israeli-Egyptian Seven Day War fails to replicate some earlier findings (Blank 1994), such differences support a view that the experience of pain varies according to cultural and historical changes. The International Association for the Study of Pain (IASP)—the major scientific organization devoted to the subject—insists that a mere transmission of nociceptive impulses does not constitute pain. In its important publication "Pain Terms" (1979), the IASP specifies that "activity induced in the nociceptor and nociceptive pathways by a noxious stimulus is not pain, which is always a psychological state . . ."

Human pain, that is, although usually associated with the activity of nociceptive impulses, requires chiefly the presence of a conscious individual perceiving mind. Pain, writes the IASP, is "always subjective." If you shut off the individual perceiving mind through sleep or anesthesia, the pain disappears. Indeed, you don't need a painful stimulus to create pain. As thousands of amputees know who suffer from phantom-limb pain, you don't even need a leg to feel pain in your leg. All you need, along with the appropriate neurobiological patterns, is a conscious mind. In a study at the Baylor College of Medicine, one hundred paid volunteers were told that the stimulus they received from an electrical stimulator might possibly create a headache (Bayer, Baer, and Early 1991). They were not told that researchers had set the stimulator so that it could not possibly produce a painful stimulus. Fifty percent of the volunteers reported pain. A similar phenomenon appears in "couvade syndrome," when the male partners of pregnant women undergo various symptoms of pregnancy, including abdominal pain (Cavenar and Weddington 1978).

The crucial importance of culture and meaning is especially vivid in the case of chronic pain. Ranjan Roy (1992) offers a scrupulous review of current research showing how chronic pain sweeps into its domain such nonbiological contributing causes as family conflict, economic stress, and a history of emotional trauma. The benefits reaped from such social forces as a disability payment or a suddenly attentive spouse can help transform a local injury—a slip in the shower or a whiplash accident—into a pain that is intractable and endless. The roots of chronic pain sometimes extend into a distant (real or imagined) past. Women suffering from irritable bowel syndrome, where an organic cause is not clear, proved significantly more likely than women with organic inflammatory bowel disease to report a history of severe life-time sexual victimization (Walker et al. 1993).

One way to see how pain entangles itself with meaning and belief is to glance at the history of art. The statue known as the Laocoön group, which ranks among the most famous works from the Greco-Roman world, shows pain absorbed into the context of tragic suffering where defeat and destruction nevertheless reveal a larger-than-life, even heroic, nobility of spirit. Christian art displays various complex readings of pain, from the vividly lacerated flesh of Matthias Grünewald's fifteenth-century Christ (whose agony marks his humanness) to Guido Reni's seventeenth-century placid and semierotic martyrdom of Saint Sebastian (whose upraised eyes link pain with the theological state called beatific vision). Such representations are not decorative artifacts but implicit or explicit guides to conduct. The ways in which a culture represents pain has much to do with how people will experience it.

One problem with this approach, which I pursue at length in *The Culture of Pain* (Morris 1991), is that skeptics can dismiss such examples as prescientific. Religious or ethical meanings, they would argue, are exactly what research has effectively dissolved by showing us the hidden neurobiology of our pain-transmission systems. In this demystified vision, nonmedical beliefs about the cultural meanings of pain belong to the benighted world before Darvon and Demerol and Dilaudid. Such a view, however, ignores the ways in which our experience of pain has been reshaped by such powerful cultural forces as drug companies and research grants. Moreover, the claim that pain is wholly meaningless remains not a fact but a belief. It also ignores the accumulating biomedical evidence that pain is still deeply influenced by what we believe.

How we think about our pain, in other words, matters greatly. The ancient Babylonians attributed headaches to an assault by malign demons. We may dismiss this belief as false, but it surely had an impact on the pain experienced by ancient Babylonians. In the nineteenth century, Dorothy Wordsworth wrote that pain was "precious" to the humble soul—because it was sent by God to remove wayward thoughts. Meaning is so important to pain that it, in some cases, can impede recovery. It is well-known that litigation and disability payments will profoundly complicate efforts at medical treatment (Mendelson 1992). On the other hand, even a belief that pain means nothing—if it replaces, say, a belief that the pain signified terminal cancer—can have an enormous impact. Like a zero in mathematics, it is very different to signify nothing than to be without meaning. Meaninglessness simply blocks the mind and shuts off a potent resource for therapy. As the current president of the IASP puts it, "All sensory phenomenon, including nociception, can be altered by conscious or unconscious mental processes" (Loeser 1991).

The mind's role in the construction of meanings for pain—even the zero degree of meaning that pain signifies nothing—has in recent years become clear through cross-cultural studies, interethnic studies, psychological studies, and studies of pain-beliefs (Morris 1995). If meaning and culture play a role in pain, for example, it follows that pain should differ across cultures. One group of researchers studied low-back patients in the United States and New Zealand, concluding that

American patients used more medication, were more likely to receive pretreatment compensation, and experienced greater "emotional and behavioral disruption" (Carron, DeGood, and Tait 1985). A similar comparison of Japanese and American low-back patients found that Japanese patients were significantly less impaired in "psychological, social, vocational, and avocational functioning" (Brena, Sanders, and Motoyama 1990). Another study comparing low-back patients in America, Japan, Mexico, Colombia, Italy, and New Zealand again found that American patients were "clearly most dysfunctional" (Sanders et al. 1992). Dysfunction here is not a separable reaction *to* pain, as if pain were the stimulus and dysfunction the response. Instead, pain comes to *include* the culturally created and reinforced meaning that a person is dysfunctional. The impact of culture is in fact so strong that a study of Anglo-Americans and native Puerto Ricans found that the two groups simply appear to experience chronic pain differently (Bates 1995).

A parallel line of study, beginning with Mark Zborowski's important book *People in Pain* (1969), shows that different ethnic groups experience pain quite differently. The specific ethnic groups that Zborowski studied—Italians, Jews, Irish, and what he called Old Americans (or, slang, WASPS)—turn out to experience a pain as distinctive as their cuisine. Even stoic denial has implications about what we believe pain signifies: for the Irish laborer it means he's out of work. Indeed, there is considerable research backing up Zborowski's general approach (Wolff and Langley 1968; Lipton and Marbach, 1984). *The Nuprin Pain Report* (1985) finds that second and third generation Americans are more likely than their first generation counterparts to report suffering from headaches, backaches, muscle pains, and stomach pains. Another study detects significant variance among ethnic groups in the "affective" dimension of pain (Greenwald 1991). Still other researchers conclude that variations in pain intensity may be affected by "attitudes, beliefs and emotional and psychological states" associated with particular ethnic groups (Bates, Edwards, Anderson 1993; Wolff 1985).

The force of such studies increases when we look at research broadly classified as psychological. Ever since publication of *The Psychology of Pain* (1978), edited by Richard A. Sternbach and now in a second edition, it has become routine to associate chronic pain with emotional states such as fear, loss, and anger. Although the specific link has proved hard to pin down, comorbidity between depression and chronic pain runs high, with some 50 percent of chronic pain patients displaying significant levels of depression (Romano and Turner 1985). Perhaps not surprisingly, tricyclic antidepressants are effective in treating a wide range of chronic pain patients (Max et al. 1991). Beyond depression, the impetus for much psychological research on pain doubtless comes from George L. Engel's classic study "'Psychogenic' Pain and the Pain Prone Patient" (1959). In his clinically based analysis, Engel found that so-called "pain prone" patients tended to be individuals for whom psychological conditions during childhood—often centering on punishment—create a template for adult experiences of pain and suffering. Clearly, some people feel driven to inflict pain or to seek it (Califa 1982; Favazza 1987). The English word *pain,* of course, derives directly from the Latin word for punishment, and it is no surprise that people who feel an extreme desire for discipline or penance eventually find their way to pain.

Studies in the personal and social psychology of pain radiate in so many directions that it is easy to ignore the central concern that they share with mind and meaning. Take, for example, the malady now called somatization disorder, in which the most common symptom (among multiple complaints that cannot be traced to tissue damage) is pain. Women vastly outnumber men among its sufferers, and the origin of such shifty pain may be circuitous or impossible to pin down. Professor of psychiatry G. Richard Smith (1991) in his book-length study of somatization disorder cites research showing that a large percentage of women with pelvic or abdominal pain report childhood incidents of sexual abuse. Even a diagnosis may mitigate or aggravate pain. Thus patients diagnosed with arthritis report significantly less pain than patients diagnosed with myofascial disorder—the latter a condition whose cause and status are still somewhat ambiguous (Faucett and Levine 1991). Pain originating in demonstrable tissue damage can be exacerbated by events that are largely mental and emotional. Anger and so-called "negative cognitions," especially punishing responses from family members, have been shown to increase pain in a condition as undeniably organic as spinal cord injury (Summers et al. 1991).

Psychological research into what are called "pain beliefs" offers a wealth of support for a biocultural model. Whatever their different schools of thought, psychologists usually agree on the basic point that pain always involves learning (Fordyce 1974). Some may disagree violently whether what is learned should be called behaviors or beliefs, but many pain specialists now take the sensible position that learning about pain extends to *both* behaviors and beliefs (Turk et al. 1983). Even pure behaviorist techniques prove effective in treating pain, it is argued, precisely because such patients develop—even if unknowingly—"new thinking skills" (Ciccone and Grzesiak 1984).

Knowledge about a patient's specific pain beliefs is useful especially because it allows therapists to anticipate problems in treatment and to help each patient develop a personalized coping strategy (Schüssler 1992). For example, David A. Williams (1989; 1991) examines what he calls "core beliefs" about pain, which involve issues of self-blame, cause, and duration. Core beliefs, he argues, predict pain intensity. Mark Jensen (1991; 1992) finds that patients function better who believe that they have some control over their pain, who believe in the value of medical services, who believe that family members care for them, and who believe that they are not severely disabled. Another study of one hundred patients shows that pain beliefs correlate directly with treatment outcomes (Shutty, DeGood, Tuttle 1990; DeGood and Shutty 1992).

It has been important here to establish and emphasize the ironclad bond between pain and belief because placebos hold serious implications for pain management (Peck and Coleman 1991) and because for over two hundred years the best scientific minds have steadfastly ignored or denied the bond between what we think and how we feel. Indeed, resistance continues to this day. The dominant medical model of pain has focused all its explanatory power on the action of nerves and neurotransmitters, to the utter exclusion of mind and culture. Only within the past few years has the dogma begun to slip and scattered researchers begun to acknowledge the impact of beliefs on pain (Helman 1984). The boldest assertions by the IASP subcommittee on nosology occur only in the footnotes to its published definition of pain. The crucial importance of belief, of course, is what links pain with placebos and (I would argue) what makes placebos so effective in the relief of pain. Placebos work not just because the nervous system has provided humans with their own endogenous pain-killing neuropeptides but because, in effect, belief proves especially effective in helping to unravel what belief has helped to construct.

Several researchers have explored the strong connection between the placebo effect and faith healing among religious sects (Plotkin 1985; Csordas 1988), but placebos do not just unravel preexisting conditions such as pain or gastric ulcers. Placebos can create problems as well as undo them. About 50 percent of experimental subjects who received placebo alcohol, for example, reported feeling slightly drunk (Hammersley, Finnigan, and Millar 1992). Some conditions are far more worrisome. One extreme example of a so-called nocebo effect—sometimes called "toxic placebos" for their power to cause harm—is voodoo death, when a healthy person who believes in sorcery dies after the proper application of a curse (Hahn and Kleinman 1983). Whether you believe you are drinking alcohol or living perilously under a witch doctor's malediction, it is culture as well as neurobiology that together constitute the matrix from which the corresponding bodily changes proceed.

Medicine as a cultural practice generates in doctors and patients a powerful set of connected beliefs that underlie any therapeutic encounter. The belief that doctors understand illness gives many patients an automatic expectation of relief such that the mere appearance of someone in a white coat—or other potent cultural image of medicine—can produce a placebo effect. In ways both subtle and diffuse, we learn to recognize the cultural signs that promise relief, from aspirin bottles to surgery. Further, most people recognize and consume medical care only within the larger context of a cultural situation in which some are designated patients and others healers. The placebo effect thus belongs to an encompassing cultural narrative in which humans project their own self-healing powers onto a doctor or shaman or priest, who triggers relief through certain arcane rituals and prescriptions. Despite the progress of modern biomedicine, it is a narrative that has not changed for thousands of years.

It seems likely that within several decades the question of how placebos work will be answered by researchers in neurobiology; but equally fascinating from the perspective of a biocultural approach is the unasked question of *why* they work. Why, that is, should humans possess the power implicit in the placebo/nocebo effect to make themselves sick or well? Apparently nobody today has gathered the evidence required for a certain answer, and it is always possible that the placebo effect is simply a freakish, vestigial byproduct of human evolution, with no purpose whatsoever. Yet another story can be told—one in which the placebo/nocebo effect, no matter how it came into being as a feature of our nerves and tissues, offered a signal contribution to human survival. In this sense, one might suspect that it remains a part of our general biological equipment because it once played a useful cultural role in the era before scientific medicine.

The brief biocultural story that I wish to tell begins with the arrival in North America of the earliest ancestors of the Indian tribe later known as the Apaches. The exact date of their arrival is still in debate, but for my purposes we should imagine it long ago, maybe several thousand years. What matters is that these new arrivals in the American Southwest faced an unfamiliar and hostile landscape that challenged all their traditions of folk medicine. Archeological evidence suggests that hunter-gather groups in general enjoy very good health (Cohen 1989). A nomadic lifestyle and small, isolated populations prevent the infections and epidemic diseases common to sedentary city-dwellers. The ancestors of the Apaches discovered new herbs and roots to deal with the normal irritants of their rugged outdoor life, from constipation (due to alternating periods of starvation and feasting) to the common cold. Indeed, the astonishingly rich herbal medicine of the Native American peoples has contributed much to the pharmacopeia of the industrial West. In this sense, Apache medicine was similar to the medical practices of other Native American tribes (Stone 1962; Vogel 1970)—and to the practice of many Stone Age peoples (Gordon 1949).

Indian medicine men and medicine women, whose methods got them routinely dismissed by white physicians as quacks, soon established a reputation among the early European settlers in America as superb healers. They were expert at curing wounds, for example, and the so-called "Indian doctor" became a fixture in frontier medicine. It is clear, however, that medicinal benefits of herbs and potions were increased by the extraordinary healing powers communicated through the shaman (Stockel 1993). The shaman was trained in the intricate rituals that accompanied Indian medicine. These rituals sometimes involved the entire community and included dance, drums, rattles, prayers, and chants. Often masked and wrapped in animal skins, the shaman was a commanding figure: Cheyenne shaman High Wolf wore a necklace ornamented with the left-hand middle fingers of eight hostile warriors whom he had killed in battle. It is well documented that shamans and their patients believed deeply in the power of these elaborate ceremonies. (The Navajo healing ceremony called Mountain Chant stretched over nine days.) In a gesture of faith that modern medicine understands quite well, patients paid the shaman handsomely in money or goods. Although some healers grew wealthy, it was not a risk-free profession: common practice held that an unsuccessful shaman might be killed by the family of the dead patient.

From a modern perspective, it seems clear that in addition to their skill in curing wounds and in dispensing herbal remedies, Native American healers made excellent use of the placebo effect. A strong placebo effect is at least predictable because shamans and patients shared the belief that illness and healing both had a supernatural source. Among the Apaches, the shaman's power came either through a special grant from a god or through possession of a sacred object. The ceremonies and rituals had as their specific aim the exorcism of evil spirits and the invocation of protective spirits. In contrast to the academic, hands-off medicine of early modern Europe, Native American shamans ministered directly to the body of the patient, often by long and intense periods of sucking on the afflicted part. This intimate contact aimed literally to suck out the evil spirit: sometimes the shaman spat out a small stone as testimony. It is hard to attribute such cures to anything other than the placebo effect. Such traditional methods, unfortunately, were powerless against the imported epidemic contagious diseases (chiefly smallpox and tuberculosis) that decimated the Indian peoples more effectively than the U. S. Army. They were also little help against the three main terrors that faced the Apaches in their nomadic day-to-day existence: snakes, bears, and ghosts.

The powerlessness of their traditional medicine against snakes, bears, and ghosts may help to explain why Apaches, both ancient and modern, experience three unusual maladies that go under the names of snake-sickness, bear-sickness, and ghost-sickness. While many tribes used herbal and homeopathic remedies to treat minor snakebites (Stone 1962), the bite of the Southwestern prairie rattler is almost invariably fatal. Among the Apaches, merely crossing the path left by a snake was enough to bring on loathsome facial sores that required the services of a shaman who specialized in snake-sickness (Opler 1935). Similarly, any contact with a bear or its den, even touching bear fur, can among the Apaches bring on physical deformities treatable only by a specialist in bear-sickness (Stockel 1993). Ditto ghosts. Ghosts and spirits are to the Apache as real and as dangerous as bears and snakes, so they must be avoided or placated at all costs. The only effective medicine here is obviously preventive medicine. Ghost-sickness, bear-sickness, and snake-sickness would (from the perspective of Western scientific thought) all seem prime instances of the nocebo effect, just as the techniques used to cure them would seem to require placebos. Together they demonstrate the power of cultural beliefs to create illness as well as to relieve it.

No doubt ghost-sickness generates the deepest skepticism among rationalists convinced that supernatural beings do not exist. Thus it is important to emphasize that ghosts are not miscellaneous spooks but an integral part of the Native American belief system in which individual illness derives from various forms of disharmony: disharmony with gods, community, neighbors, family, animals, and earth (Perrone, Stockel, and Kreuger 1989). The chants and songs integral to most Native American healing ceremonies are images of harmony. They express the collective will to promote individual health by restoring a proper relation to the community and spirit world. Indeed, all healing among the Native American people is attributed ultimately to spiritual power. Someone who reports seeing a ghost, then, is not expressing credulity or self-deception but rather an acute sense of disharmony with the spirit world. Where life among Native Americans reserves such a central role for the on-going communal links to gods and ancestors, it is easy to imagine ghost-sickness as a paradigm of much illness in signifying that the individual has fallen out of the state of harmony necessary to health.

The burden of my biocultural tale is to suggest that early humans or hominids who had access to the placebo/nocebo effect—activated through powerful beliefs in supernatural sources of healing and ill-ness—would have secured an advantage over early people who did not. Before antibiotics, placebos and herbs were the most effective medical treatments available. Psychiatrist Arthur Shapiro has proposed that the placebo response is part of our "genetic inheritance" (Cherry 1981). It was certainly useful that the Apaches possessed in the nocebo effect a biological means to promote an avoidance of bears and snakes, just as Apache culture possessed in the placebo effect a way to undo the sickness apparently caused by snakes and bears and ghosts. The several million years needed to trace the development of early humans has not yet provided good evidence about the evolutionary origin of the pla-cebo effect. Such evidence would likely involve complex applications of "gene-culture coevolution" (Lumsden and Wilson 1985) and "biologi-cally prepared learning" (Ulrich 1993). It would also need to explain why some people apparently lose or never possess the power of re-sponding to placebos. The main point, regardless, remains secure. Illness and healing, while they clearly require a neurobiology, require a culture as well, because cultures provide both the material conditions (from sickbeds to toxic dumps) and the immaterial beliefs that directly affect human health. Indeed, a culture so powerfully shapes and modifies our experience that individuals always reflect, even if they resist, its influence. It is in this sense that a full theory of placebo will necessarily be biocultural (McElroy 1990).

A biocultural model, of course, must include whatever we can learn about the neurobiology of analgesia, conditioning, and symptom relief. Yet neurobiology will never encompass the whole event. An adequate model must acknowledge the ways in which the human nervous system is set into motion by the impact of mind and culture. Indeed, such interaction helps explain why the long-term failure of medical treat-ment has been shown capable of suppressing and extinguishing the placebo response (White et al. 1985). A biocultural model remains at present a conceptual tool: we do not yet know enough details. Yet, this uncomfortable point is exactly where placebos may have their most important function. In demanding a model that goes beyond cultural or biological explanations alone, placebos insist on a comprehensive explanatory vision that amounts almost to a new way of thinking. The way of thinking that I recommend here sees human bodies not as

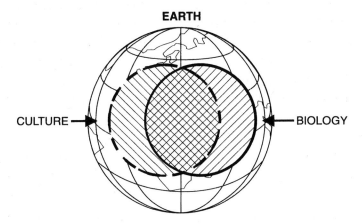

Figure 9.1 Human beings and complex human events are constructed at the intersection of culture and biology

biological mechanisms independent of mind and culture; it sees the person not as a self-contained psychic unit independent of culture or body. Rather, it regards human beings and complex human events like health and illness as constructed at the intersection of culture and biology.

Diagrams obviously oversimplify. The broken circles in Figure 9.1 are meant to indicate that the boundaries are permeable and shifty. The cross-hatching indicates that the earth—as opposed to the anthropocentric world of belief systems and skyscrapers that we scratch upon its surface (Heidegger 1971)—contains much that eludes us, that resists and withholds explanation, that withdraws into silence, reserved and incommunicable. Our biology, like our cultures, limits the world that we recognize, much as we cannot hear low or high frequencies audible to elephants and dogs. Moreover, we still reflect in our psychology the experience of prehuman ancestors who moved in an environment where nature, not culture, was the primary force that shaped them (Kaplan and Kaplan 1989). Despite its limitations, however, a biocultural view is simply more accurate in accounting for pain and for the placebo effect than are biological or cultural explanations alone.

Placebos, ever since they joined the medical lexicon in 1811, have been considered mostly a nuisance—or worse—because they just didn't fit within the borders of a mechanical model. Like a wedge, they may now help finally shatter a mechanistic view of human life. The transition to new ways of thinking is difficult, not least because cultures embroil us in mixed or contradictory meanings, a situation which not only complicates the understanding of pain (Johnson 1989) but also introduces into biocultural studies the messy variables that scientific research usually tries so hard to exclude. A biocultural model is no panacea, but it promises to evoke studies that cannot simply resemble the monologues of separate disciplines, no matter how powerful or prestigious. The challenge of placebos to contemporary thought is whether they demand not just another explanatory mechanism (keyed to the old medical model) but a new, dialogical vision that sees culture as indelibly influenced by human biology and that sees human biology as deeply engaged and even modified by the shaping influence of culture.

References

Archer, Thomas P., and Carl V. Leier. 1992. "Placebo Treatment in Congestive Heart Failure." *Cardiology,* 81:125–133.

Bates, Maryann S., W. Thomas Edwards, and Karen O. Anderson. 1993. "Ethnocultural Influences on Variation in Chronic Pain Perception." *Pain,* 52:101–112.

Bates, Maryann S., L. Rankin-Hill, M. Sanchez-Ayendez, and R. Mendez-Bryan. 1995. "A Cross-Cultural Comparison of Adaptation to Chronic Pain Among Anglo-Americans and Native Puerto Ricans." *Medical Anthropology,* 16:141–173.

Bayer, Timothy L., Paul E. Baer, and Charles Early. 1991. "Situational and Psychophysiological Factors in Psychologically Induced Pain." *Pain,* 44:45–50.

Beecher, Henry K. 1946. "Pain in Men Wounded in Battle." *The Bulletin of the U.S. Army Medical Department,* 5:445–454.

Benson, Herbert, and David P. McCallie, Jr. 1979. "Angina Pectoris and the Placebo Effect." *New England Journal of Medicine,* 300:1424–1429.

Blank, Jon W. 1994. "Pain in Men Wounded in Battle: Beecher Revisited." *IASP Newsletter,* January/February:2–4.

Brena, Steven F., Steven H. Sanders, and Hiroshi Motoyama. 1990. "American and Japanese Chronic Low Back Pain Patients: Cross-Cultural Similarities and Differences." *The Clinical Journal of Pain,* 6:118–124.

Brown, Walter A., Mary F. Johnson, and Mon-Gy Chen. 1992. "Clinical

Features of Depressed Patients Who Do and Do Not Improve With Placebo." *Psychiatry Research,* 41:203–214.

Califa, Pat. 1982. "Feminism and Sadomasochism." *The CoEvolution Quarterly,* 33 (Spring):33–40.

Carron, Harold, Douglas E. DeGood, and Raymond Tait. 1985. "A Comparison of Low Back Pain Patients in the United States and New Zealand: Psychosocial and Economic Factors Affecting Severity of Disability." *Pain,* 21:77–89.

Cavenar, Jesse O., Jr., and William W. Weddington, Jr. 1978. "Abdominal Pain in Expectant Fathers." *Psychosomatics,* 19:761–768.

Cherry, Laurence. 1981. "The Power of the Empty Pill." *Science Digest,* 89 (8):60–62, 67, 116.

Ciccone, Donald S., and Roy C. Grzesiak. 1984. "Cognitive Dimensions of Chronic Pain." *Social Science and Medicine,* 19:1339–1345.

Cohen, Mark Nathan. 1989. *Health and the Rise of Civilization.* New Haven: Yale University Press.

Csordas, Thomas J. 1988. "Elements of Charismatic Persuasion and Healing." *Medical Anthropology Quarterly,* 2:121–142.

DeGood, Douglas E., and Michael S. Shutty, Jr. 1992. "Assessment of Pain Beliefs, Coping, and Self-Efficacy." *Handbook of Pain Assessment.* ed. Dennis C. Turk and Ronald Melzack. New York: Guilford Press, p. 214–234.

Engel, George L. 1959. "'Psychogenic' Pain and the Pain-Prone Patient." *American Journal of Medicine,* 26:899–918.

Faucett, Julia A., and Jon D. Levine. 1991. "The Contributions of Interpersonal Conflict to Chronic Pain in the Presence or Absence of Organic Pathology." *Pain,* 44:35–43.

Favazza, Armando R., with Barbara Favazza. 1987. *Bodies Under Siege: Self-mutilation in Culture and Psychiatry.* Baltimore, Md.: Johns Hopkins University Press.

Fordyce, Wilbert E. 1974. "Pain Viewed as Learned Behavior." *Advances in Neurology.* Vol. 4. ed. John J. Bonica. New York: Raven Press, p. 415–422.

Foucault, Michel. 1973. *The Birth of the Clinic: An Archaeology of Medical Perception* (1963). trans. A. M. Sheridan Smith. New York: Pantheon Books.

Gordon, Benjamin Lee. 1949. *Medicine Throughout Antiquity.* Philadelphia: F. A. Davis.

Greenwald, Howard P. 1991. "Interethnic Differences in Pain Perception." *Pain,* 44:157–163.

Hahn, Robert A., and Arthur Kleinman. 1983. "Belief as Pathogen, Belief as Medicine: 'Voodoo Death' and the 'Placebo Phenomenon' in Anthropological Perspective." *Medical Anthropology Quarterly,* 14 (4):3, 16–19.

Hammersley, Richard, Frances Finnigan, and Keith Millar. 1992. "Alcohol Placebos: You Can Only Fool Some of the People All of the Time." *British Journal of Addiction,* 87:1477–1480.

Hashish, Ibrahim, H. Hai, W. Harvey, C. Feinmann, and M. Harris. 1988. "Reduction of Postoperative Pain and Swelling by Ultrasound Treatment: A Placebo Effect." *Pain,* 33:303–311.

Heidegger, Martin. 1971. "The Origin of the Work of Art" (1935). *Poetry, Language, Thought.* Trans. Albert Hofstader. New York: Harper & Row. p. 15–87.

Helman, Cecil. 1984. "Pain and Culture." *Culture, Health and Illness: An Introduction for Health Professionals.* Bristol: John Wright & Sons, p. 95–105.

IASP Subcommittee on Taxonomy Pain Terms. "Pain Terms: A List with Definitions and Notes on Usage." 1979. *Pain,* 6:249–252.

Jensen, Mark P., J. A. Turner, J. M. Romano, and P. Karoly. 1991. "Coping With Chronic Pain: A Critical Review of the Literature." *Pain,* 47:249–283.

Jensen, Mark P., and Paul Karoly. 1992. "Pain-Specific Beliefs, Perceived Symptom Severity, and Adjustment to Chronic Pain." *The Clinical Journal of Pain,* 8:123–130.

Johnson, Thomas M. 1989. "Contradictions in the Cultural Construction of Pain in America." *Advances in Pain Research and Therapy.* Vol. 11. C. Stratton Hill, Jr. and William S. Fields, eds. New York: Raven Press, p. 27–37.

Kaplan, Rachel, and Stephen Kaplan. 1989. *The Experience of Nature: A Psychological Perspective.* New York: Cambridge University Press.

Levine, Jon D., Newton C. Gordon, and Howard L. Fields. 1978. "The Mechanism of Placebo Analgesia." *Lancet* 2:654–657.

Lipton, James A., and Joseph J. Marbach. 1984. "Ethnicity and the Pain Experience." *Social Science and Medicine,* 19:1279–1298.

Loeser, John D. 1991. "What Is Chronic Pain?" *Theoretical Medicine,* 12:213–225.

Lumsden, Charles J., and Edward O. Wilson. 1985 [1958]. "The Relation Between Biological and Cultural Evolution." *Journal of Social and Biological Structure,* 8:343–359.

Mavissakalian, Matig R., Bruce Jones, and Stephen Olson. 1990. "Absence of Placebo Response in Obsessive-Compulsive Disorder." *Journal of Nervous and Mental Diseases,* 178:268–270.

Max, Mitchell B., R. Kishore-Kumar, S. C. Schafer, B. Meister, R. H. Gracely, B. Smoller, and R. Dubner. 1991. "Efficacy of Desipramine in Painful Diabetic Neuropathy: A Placebo-controlled Trial." *Pain,* 45:3–9.

McElroy, Ann. 1990. "Biocultural Models in Studies of Human Health and Adaptation." *Medical Anthropology Quarterly,* 4:243–265.

Melzack, Ronald. 1960. "The Personal Pain." *Essays of Our Time I.* Leo Hamalian and Edmond L. Volpe, ed. New York: McGraw Hill, p. 172–177.

Mendelson, George. 1992. "Compensation and Chronic Pain." *Pain,* 48:121–123.

Moerman, Daniel E. 1983. "General Medical Effectiveness and Human Biology: Placebo Effects in the Treatment of Ulcer Disease." *Medical Anthropology Quarterly,* 14 (4):3, 13–16.

Morris, David B. 1991. *The Culture of Pain.* Berkeley: University of California Press.

———. 1995. "What We Make of Pain." *The Wilson Quarterly,* 18 (4):8–26.

The Nuprin Pain Report. 1985. New York: Louis Harris and Associates.

Opler, M. E. 1935. "The Concept of Supernatural Power Among the Chiricahua and Mescalero Apaches." *American Anthropologist,* 37:65–70.

Peck, Connie, and Grahame Coleman. 1991. "Implications of Placebo Theory for Clinical Research and Practice in Pain Management." *Theoretical Medicine,* 12:247–270.

Perrone, Bobette, H. Henrietta Stockel, and Victoria Krueger. 1989. *Medicine Women, "Curanderas," and Women Doctors.* Norman: University of Oklahoma Press.

Plotkin, William B. 1985. "A Psychological Approach to Placebo: The Role of Faith in Therapy and Treatment." *Placebo: Theory, Research, and Mechanisms.* Leonard White, Bernard Tursky, and Gary E. Schwartz, eds. New York: Guilford Press, p. 237–254.

Raftery, E. B., and B. A. Gould. 1990. "The Effect of Placebo on Indirect and Direct Blood Pressure Measurements." *Journal of Hypertension,* 8 (6):S93-S100.

Romano, Joan M., and Judith A. Turner. 1985. "Chronic Pain and Depression: Does the Evidence Support a Relationship?" *Psychological Bulletin,* 97:18–34.

Roy, Ranjan. 1992. *The Social Context of the Chronic Pain Sufferer.* Toronto: University of Toronto Press.

Sanders, Steven H., S. F. Brena, C. J. Spier, D. Beltrutti, H. McConnell, and O. Quintero. 1992. "Chronic Low Back Pain Patients Around the World: Cross-Cultural Similarities and Differences." *The Clinical Journal of Pain,* 8:317–323.

Scarry, Elaine. 1985. *The Body in Pain: The Making and Unmaking of the World.* New York: Oxford University Press.

Schüssler, Gerhard. 1992. "Coping Strategies and Individual Meanings of Illness." *Social Science and Medicine,* 34:427–432.

Shutty, Michael S., Jr., Douglas E. DeGood, and Diane H. Tuttle. 1990. "Chronic Pain Patients' Beliefs About Their Pain and Treatment

Outcomes." *Archives of Physical Medicine and Rehabilitation*, 71:128–132.

Smith, G. Richard, Jr. 1991. *Somatization Disorder in the Medical Setting*. Washington, D.C.: American Psychiatric Press.

Sternbach, Richard A. ed. *The Psychology of Pain*. 1986. 2nd edn. New York: Raven Press.

Stockel, H. Henrietta. 1993. *Survival of the Spirit: Chiricahua Apaches in Captivity*. Reno: University of Nevada Press.

Stone, Eric. 1962. *Medicine Among the American Indians*. New York: Hafner.

Summers, Jay D., M. A. Rapoff, G. Varghese, K. Porter, and R. E. Palmer. 1991. "Psychosocial Factors in Chronic Spinal Cord Injury Pain." *Pain,* 47:183–189.

Thomas, K. B. 1987. "General Practice Consultations: Is There Any Point in Being Positive?" *British Medical Journal,* 294:1200–1202.

Turk, Dennis C., Donald Meichenbaum, and Myles Genest. 1983. *Pain and Behavioral Medicine: A Cognitive-Behavioral Perspective*. New York: Guilford Press.

Turner, Judith A., R. A. Deyo, J. D. Loeser, Michael Von Korff, and Wilbert E. Fordyce. 1994. "The Importance of Placebo Effects in Pain Treatment and Research." *JAMA,* 271:1609–1614.

Ulrich, Roger S. 1993. "Biophilia, Biophobia, and Natural Landscapes." *The Biophilia Hypothesis*. Stephen R. Kellert and Edward O. Wilson, eds. Washington, D.C.: Island Press, p. 73–137.

Vogel, Virgil J. 1970. *American Indian Medicine*. Norman: University of Oklahoma Press.

Voudouris, Nicholas J., Connie L. Peck, and Grahame Coleman. 1989. "Conditioned Response Models of Placebo Phenomena: Further Support." *Pain* 38:109–116.

Walker, Edward A., W. J. Katon, P. P. Roy-Byrne, R. P. Jemelka, and J. Russo. 1993. "Histories of Sexual Victimization in Patients With Irritable Bowel Syndrome or Inflammatory Bowel Disease." *American Journal of Psychiatry,* 150:1502–1506.

Wall, Patrick D. 1992. "The Placebo Effect: An Unpopular Topic." *Pain,* 51:1–3.

———. 1993. "Pain and the Placebo Response." *Ciba Foundation Symposium,* 174:187–211; discussion 212–216.

White, L., B. Turskey, and G. E. Schwartz, eds. 1985. *Placebo: Theory, Research, and Mechanisms*. New York: Guildford Press.

Williams, David A., and Francis J. Keefe. 1991. "Pain Beliefs and the Use of Cognitive-behavioral Coping Strategies." *Pain,* 46:185–190.

Williams, David A., and Beverly E. Thorn. 1989. "An Empirical Assessment of Pain Beliefs." *Pain,* 36:351–358.

Wolff, B. Berthold. 1985. "Ethnocultural Factors Influencing Pain and Illness Behavior." *The Clinical Journal of Pain,* 1:23–30.

Wolff, B. Berthold, and Sarah Langley. 1968. "Cultural Factors and the Response to Pain: A Review." *American Anthropologist,* 70:494–501.

Zborowski, Mark. 1969. *People in Pain.* San Francisco: Jossey-Bass.

Placebo: Conversations at the Disciplinary Borders

Edited by Anne Harrington

Dialogue Participants

Robert Ader, George L. Engle Professor of Psychosocial Medicine and Director of the Division of Behavioral and Psychosocial Medicine in the Department of Psychiatry at the University of Rochester School of Medicine and Dentistry.

Arthur Barsky, Professor of Psychiatry, Harvard University Medical School.

Herbert Benson, Professor of Medicine, Harvard Medical School; Chief of the Division of Behavioral Medicine, Deaconess Hospital; President, Mind/Body Medical Institute.

Allan Brandt, Professor of the History of Science, Harvard University; Amalie Moses Kass Professor of the History of Medicine, Harvard Medical School.

Howard Brody, Professor of Family Practice and Philosophy and Director of the Center for Ethics and Humanities in the Life Sciences, Michigan State University.

Howard L. Fields, Professor of Neurobiology and Physiology, University of California, San Francisco.

Anne Harrington, Professor of the History of Science, Harvard University.

Kenneth Hugdahl, Department of Biological and Medical Psychology, Somatic Psychology, University of Bergen, Norway.

Steven Hyman, Director of the National Institute of Mental Health,

208

Bethesda, Maryland; Associate Professor of Psychiatry and Neuroscience, Harvard Medical School.

Michael Jensen, Edsel Bryant Ford Professor of Business Administration, Harvard Business School.

Gordon Kaufman, Mallinckrodt Professor of Divinity, Emeritus, Harvard University.

Irving Kirsch, Professor of Psychology, University of Connecticut.

Arthur Kleinman, The Maude and Lillian Presely Professor of Medical Anthropology and Psychology, Harvard University.

Stephen Kosslyn, Professor of Psychology, Harvard University.

Godehard Oepen, Associate Professor of Psychiatry, Boston University, Bedford V. A. Hospital.

Donald D. Price, Professor and Director of Research Anesthesiology, Medical College of Virginia.

Robert Rose, Director of Health Program, Mind-Body Interactions, MacArthur Foundation.

Elaine Scarry, Professor of English in American Literature, Harvard University.

Howard Spiro, Professor of Medicine and Director of the Program for Humanities in Medicine, Yale School of Medicine.

Alan Stone, Toureff-Glueck Professor of Law and Psychiatry in the Faculty of Law and the Faculty of Medicine, Harvard University.

"Body" Pain versus "Soul" Pain

Spiro: I gave up doing endoscopies in about 1968 because I really wasn't interested in using my hands anymore to find out what was going on with people. I wanted to use my ears. As a result, I tend to see more and more patients who just have pain, and so I think a lot about *why* they have pain, about the meaning of their pain. And I have concluded that there are really two fundamental kinds of pain, which demand different kinds of responses from us physicians. There are patients with acute pain, whom we physicians love to treat. You go into a case like that feeling like a knight, very macho, because you know that acute pain means tissue damage that will have a locus you are going to find and be able to do something about. You can always come up with the answer to acute pain.

So-called chronic pain, however, is a different story. One of the major problems in treating it is that it may or may not be pain. It may be suffering, mental anguish, as C. S. Lewis suggested—what I call "existential pain." I saw a woman about three weeks ago who had nausea, fullness, a little pain—clearly the kind of symptoms that make a physician's spirits sink because you know, again, you are never going to come up with the answer. She was about thirty-four years of age, married with children. As I talked with her, it turned out that the pain had started on Mother's Day two years before. She had been moving up the ladder in her corporation, a Fortune 500 company, but because her husband was also moving up a different ladder, she decided two years before that it was her job to stay home with the kids. I didn't give her any placebos—I talk about them more than I use them. But you know, that sort of thing needs some help. Maybe the psychiatrist would say that understanding is enough, but I'm not sure that it really is. It certainly hasn't been in her case so far.

Harrington: I was thinking that, for many people in our society, it is not particularly acceptable to seek help from a doctor or a healer because you have existential anguish. But it is acceptable to seek help because you have got an ulcer. In this sense, a patient can come to a doctor and use the language of the body, the language of "pain" to talk about his or her existential anguish; and placebos may be one way that doctors can respond to patients, with an intervention that appears also to be "just" about the body and "just" about pain. But at the same time there may be a whole different level of conversation going on somewhere under the surface.

Spiro: You are saying, in a sense, that we doctors are more elitist than we like to pretend, that we are dealing with a patient who comes in to us and says, "I have pain." *We* know that pain is anguish, *we* know that pain is something else, but we don't really address it on that level, we still deal with it as pain. Is that what you are saying?

Harrington: No, I wasn't thinking so much about an elitist agenda, as much as reflecting on the possibility that in our society, the language of the body, of physical disease, is the most acceptable language we have to talk about suffering.

"Illnesses" versus "Diseases"

Spiro: As a biomedical physician, I like to discriminate between the disease, which is what the physician or the imaging technologies can detect, and the illness, what the patient feels. For me, as a gastroenterologist, disease is the stomach ulcer; dyspepsia, its pain, is the illness. And it is important to realize that there is no tight relationship, no tight relationship at all, between the presence of an ulcer crater and the presence of dyspepsia.

From experience, I know that placebos can do a lot for dyspepsia, but there isn't really, so near as I can see, a shred of evidence that placebos alter the course of what I call disease. I know that flies against the trend of the times, and I worry when I say it because people really want to believe that they can control all sorts of things. But my usual reply is, well, you can help the pain of cancer, but I'm not really sure you can help cancer in any other way.

The analogy I use, is of a stream flowing by someone's backyard. It is very easy to dam it up when there is very little water there. When that stream is converted into a torrent, when there is water coming down from Sleeping Giant, in Hamden, or when the Mississippi River is swollen over its banks, you can't stop that. That's why I always say to myself, it's too bad that people who are fatally ill are made to feel doubly bad—not only are they dying and unable to stop the process, but they are also being told that they should be able to stop something unstoppable, by visualizing their cells doing one thing or another.

Rose: I wonder if I might push you a little bit to unpack this metaphor of the stream behind the house. It seems that you are suggesting that the placebo effect is alive and well, i.e., functionally active, in the domains of symptomatology that people experience, like fatigue, depression, demoralization, and, of course, pain. On the other hand, you say that there is very little evidence, and I think you're right, that placebos can affect the course of diseases, like neoplasm and cancers, which are run amok. We have a handful of anecdotes, single case examples, where it seems like effects have been shown, tumors have regressed and so on, but we don't know how good the evidence is, or really very much about that.

What I'm curious about instead is the world of clinical change we might imagine exists "in-between" pure symptomatology on the one hand, and full-blown disease on the other. Studies have been carried out in which individuals who took a cholesterol-lowering drug were compared with a placebo control, and it was found that the magnitude in the fall of cholesterol was equivalent in those two groups among those individuals who took the pills religiously, regardless of whether they were taking an active drug or a placebo. The "active" factor here seemed to be compliance or adherence to the treatment. So, here we have something which is in between, as it were: physiological changes that have clear health implications resulting from placebo treatment.

Spiro: Well, I'd like to have Herbert Benson respond to this, since he has done a lot of work with hypertension and a lot of other kinds of things in that in-between area you refer to. What about it?

Benson: Well, I was going to actually ask you a question, and it picks up on something which Bob Rose has just touched on. Where in your thinking does the line between disease and illness intersect? I think most would agree that the rampant neoplasm is going to be very little altered by placebo effects. Yet irritable bowel syndrome may well be. But what about that middle zone? What diseases would you include where there is a component both of disease and of illness and what are your opinions, relative to the affects of placebo in that middle ground?

Spiro: Let me turn that question back to you, since you have done so much work in hypertension. As a disorder, it seems ready-made for your own question: is that a disease, or is that a physiological response?

Benson: Our answer to that is really to simply beg the question: we say, to the extent that a disorder is stress-related—which, by your criteria, would make them illnesses but not diseases—then to that extent, mind-body therapies have applicability. But we cannot predict which patients are going to respond to those therapies. So, what we do is work with a multifaceted therapeutic package and get results, but we can't say this much of the disorder was due to the illnesses that the mind imposes on the body, this much was due to heredity, and this much was due to a sensitivity to sodium, let's say. So I am very interested in this interface between illness and disease, so we could come up with the specificity you rightfully say is so important.

Scarry: Is it possible that, to some extent, the distinction between "disease" and "illness" is circular, because we make the distinction in part by whether or not a syndrome is susceptible to placebo effects? If something we might have been inclined to call disease seems at all responsive to psychological intervention or to reassurance or to strategies of instruction and so forth, then the lines begin to waver for us a little bit, and we are more willing to imagine that this is really a response to life rather than—

Spiro: Well, yes, I take your point. To a certain extent I can see that I am caught in my own bind of saying, "Well, if I can see it, it is a disease; if I don't see it, it's an illness." And that obviously makes it depend on the technology, and the criteria therefore may change ten, twenty, thirty years down the line. But this is where I'm currently stuck.

Scarry: It seems as though, especially if one takes into account the kind of effect that a placebo can have, say, on lowering cholesterol, definitions of what is a disease get blurry. You mentioned that in certain kinds of research on heart conditions there were certain biochemical changes that came about from placebo use. If one found some coherent and systematic way of affecting such processes through psychological means, then are we in effect transforming what once appeared to be disease into something else that we have no good way of defining? Do we have to revise our basic definitions? Don't we think of disease as something that is solidly biological and intransigent, except maybe to other kinds of biological interventions?

Spiro: I think of cancer that way. I am not sure that I think of most diseases that way. I'm an optimist because I am a gastroenterologist, and in my field, people get better most of the time.

Sullivan: On the one hand, when we talk about disease and you use these images of the water torrent, we all seem to want to hang onto some notion of intransigence, some notion of an unbending physical course with a final, inevitable outcome. Yet I was also very interested just now to hear you say that part of how "diseases" come to be defined is through the whole process of diagnosis and objectification through technology. So we're left with the question of whether, so to speak, there can be a "disease" falling in the forest with no one there to hear it. It seems to me that, if you open up that door, then there may be a whole further chain of associations that suddenly get us out of the realm of mechanism and physical intransigence, and into the realm of the spouse, who is sick of hearing her husband complain, and tells him to "Please go and see the doctor." Or, into the workplace and the patient that needs an exculpatory note. It seems to me that we're then forced to consider how far actually part of what goes into making a "disease" is the social panorama.

Spiro: I agree a hundred percent. Again, I draw these dichotomies, as many doctors do, but I agree that the border is very fuzzy.

An example I use is the woman who is a physician. She is home taking care of the kids after three o'clock in the afternoon. At seven o'clock, the garage door opens, and her somewhat disliked husband, the lawyer, is coming home, and at that point she gets abdominal pain somewhere between the diaphragm and the pubis. What can she do? Well, if she wants, she can go to a clergyman. She can also go to a lawyer. But my profession hopes that she will go to a doctor, one of any number of specialties.

Yet any of them, on hearing about the pain in this area, will immediately say, "I have got to rule out disease in my field," and won't be interested that the pain comes on when the garage door goes up. Instead, the neurologist might make a diagnosis of interstitial cystitis. The gynecologist will say, "Well, you have got endometriosis, a little bit, and you have also got a little ovarian cyst that we have got to do something about." The garage door has nothing to do with it. The gastroenterologist will find that she has slightly disordered bowel function, maybe from the garage door opening, and he or she will colonoscope the patient, put a tube all the way around to the appendix, and say you have got an irritable bowel and prescribe 25 grams of fiber every day. So what we do is convert the complaints into organic disease that we think we can deal with.

Sullivan: That is extremely helpful. Is it so, then, that the different domains of the body, for the various specialties involved, function as a classificatory schema for things that we may conclude are actually not exhaustively organic?

Spiro: Absolutely, it happens all the time.

Kosslyn: It is clear that even a so-called "functional" event has to have a physical substrate. Even as you are hearing somebody talk, there are physical changes in your brain. So, this distinction we make between functional and organic seems pretty spurious—as if the one is floating out there somewhere in space, while only the other is really grounded in physical processes.

For me the further question is, whether we know if there is a distinction between the kind of central nervous system events that we call "functional," events that underlie the phenomenological experience of "illness" that are known to respond to placebo, and more peripheral physiological events that produce effects we call "disease," events that may do things like make a hole in your stomach.

Spiro: I don't know the answer to that. That's what we're all here to try to figure out.

Fields: Well, think about this: nobody would argue that if a very large spider came into the room, there would be some kind of psychic experience that we would all have. Probably 99 percent of us in the room, if you measured, if you monitored our bodies, you could detect changes. For example, an increase in pulse rate; okay? It's physical, it's peripheral, but no one would dispute that what generated it was something that happened in your nervous system.

So, one of the ways that we could think about dealing with this would be to say that a brain circuit is a physical entity; but it can also be a representation of something going on in your body. So, for example, I pinch your finger, a circuit is activated in your brain, and you have a sensation that your finger has been pinched. You could produce a similar event by electrically stimulating that circuit. So, if someone did a craniotomy and put an electrode on your somatosensory cortex and stimulated it, you would feel some tingling in your finger, even though this sensation wasn't happening in your finger. At the level of the neural circuit, all forms of human experience, whether they are of the body or the external world, have this existence as a representation in a neural circuit.

Kosslyn: I've done a lot of Positive Emission Tomography and functional MRI with mental imagery, and I show that very similar circuits in the brain are activated when your eyes are closed and when you are visualizing something, as when you are actually seeing it. Furthermore, lots of people have shown that you get skin conductance effects and various autonomic outflow effects when you have people visualize emotional stimuli. So there clearly is a physical substrate that is activated by a thought, by an idea, and these can have an affect on peripheral physiology. If the circuitry is there, why can't the physiology of the body itself be affected by certain kinds of brain events, and result in cases where something like a placebo could alter the course of what everyone would agree is a disease?

Do We Mistake "Natural" Fluctuations in Disease State for Placebo Effects?

Fields: This might be a good time to talk about something that is very important to me: the issue of spontaneous remission of disease, and whether or not you can really observe a placebo response. Probably the biggest enemy of understanding the placebo is common sense. Common sense says, I see something happen, there was an event that preceded it. The event that preceded it caused the event to happen. But in fact, I'm going to point out that you can't really observe an individual instance of placebo response; that such conclusions are always highly inferential.

Let's look at the natural history of an experience that is familiar to all of us: a headache. You start with no pain, you go over time to peak pain, and you wind up with no pain again. Let's say you observe a thousand instances of the course of a headache, you get a standard deviation, and develop your average time course of this disorder, that may well be different for different individuals.

But let's say that you give somebody a placebo at the point just after peak pain, and right before the natural diminution of pain. Since all headaches resolve spontaneously, there will be what some people would call a 100 percent placebo response. But it's a false inference. You got better after the placebo, but there was no placebo response.

Given that, how does one then differentiate between natural history of disease and placebo effects? Only through the collectivity. If you have groups of people that have gotten a placebo and groups of people that have gotten no treatment, there will be a mean difference between them: that is your placebo effect. What you found might represent a big effect in a few people, or a small effect in a lot of people. This means that the whole idea that there is a percentage of people who are responders to placebo is unsubstanitated—it's not something you know. Yet over and over people make these sorts of claims.

Kirsch: I think the problem is a real one, but it is not, in essence, different from the problem of determining a response to any other treatment, to an active drug, to a surgical intervention. You don't see it, typically, in an individual. That's why you use the placebo control group.

Fields: Absolutely.

Kirsch: And you infer the drug response from the difference between the two. The problem is that there are very few studies in which, in addition to using the placebo control group, you have some kind of base rate, or no treatment control group. Because if you had that, you would know as much about placebos as you now know about active medications and surgical procedures.

Barsky: When we do things like talk about the natural course of these things, we always run up against an enormous sampling bias. Our whole notion of what the natural course of the disease is, is based upon people who show up in physicians' offices, and return for treatment over some period of time. We base our notion of a degenerative illness like multiple sclerosis on people like that; and we just don't know about people who have one episode and then never go back to the neurologist again. So I think this idea of comparing the placebo against a no-treatment, no-intervention group, is crucial.

Kleinman: It seems to me that Howard Field's use of language like that—diseases that follow a "natural course"—is one of the classic ways medicine has of affirming one of its fundamental ideological positions: that diseases are diatheses that are epigenetically programmed to unfold, independent of the body of the host or the context. Now, that is just plain wrong. If you look at HIV infection, for example: in the United States versus Zaire, the comparative life span from the time of diagnosis, or even from the time of the infection to death, is twice as long in the United States. And that difference has to do, not with the natural but with the social course of disease: the fact that there is malnutrition and absence of treatments interacting with an impaired immune system. Similarly, with the headache example Howard Fields gave: when do you see people, except in the laboratory, who have the natural course of a headache? People intervene in all sorts of ways when they have a headache or are in distress.

Pain and Placebo Analgesia: Mechanisms and Motivations

Fields: Pain is a great paradigm for studying the kinds of behaviors we're interested in here. First of all, it is cross-culturally universal as a human experience; we all have it, and we all pretty much know what it is. Second, it is clinically significant: it is part of almost every serious medical illness. This makes it eminently fundable when you write a grant proposal, which is also important. We presume that it is mediated by circuits that are homologous, across all mammalian species. Finally, we know that we can affect it with placebos: placebo analgesia is a very robust phenomenon.

Barsky: I think here, though, of the extent to which we see a placebo effect in nonpainful stimuli. Do you have any sense of how we might think of the mechanisms and circuits functioning in those situations—for example, when the placebo works to suppress coughing, or nausea, or shortness of breath?

Fields: I would point out that the best cough suppressants are opioids and the cough is a reflex to a noxious stimulus. I would assume that the same principles would apply. Anxiety, I think, that is also highly responsive to placebo, is something that we need to think about. But again, I would say that it is not fundamentally different in its substance than pain, and may be clinically closely related. At any rate, there is a representation for anxiety in our brain circuitry, just as there is a representation for pain. Pain is a better paradigm in a way, because we know its neuroanatomy, and we have its physiology well in hand. But I would say that it is a model that predicts that there should be other syndromes that would respond to placebos in a way that is analogous, just as you suggest.

Benson: So, Howard Fields, are you suggesting that virtually all placebo phenomena are related to endogenous opioids, or do you see room for another model?

Fields: Oh, no. I think I pretty explicitly stated that I believe there are nonopioid placebo analgesias. I don't think the opioid thing is a big deal. It is just one neurotransmitter.

Benson: Let me just hone that a bit more. Do you see placebo phenomena unrelated to pain?

Fields: Absolutely, absolutely.

Stone: Well, I need to say something here about the relationship Howard Fields is making between pain and anxiety, because I think we have a contradiction in the making here. In the clinic, we know that anxiety enhances pain; one of the key components involved in producing a placebo analgesia is to calm the patient down and say, "This is going to help you." Yet, when you talk about your experimental work, you tell us that you actually produce analgesia in animals by scaring them. How do you resolve that in your own mind? Because otherwise, I am going to be lost here while we go on.

Fields: I can sort of escape that question by saying that is what we want to study.

Stone: I see.

Fields: What I would predict is that if you had an experiment where you gave a person a pill, and said, "This is a very powerful pain reliever, take it," and so on, and then you compare the person to an untreated group, you will see a placebo effect. However, if you were to take a third group and say, "Look, this is a very powerful pain killer, but it is a dangerous drug, and I don't give it out lightly. Here is a list of potential things that could happen to you if you take it." My prediction is that the pill that is described as dangerous might be a more effective placebo. In other words, part of what we do as physicians is to scare people, and that adds to our own placebo effectiveness.

Stone: It gives a whole new sense to my bedside manner.

Harrington: On the other hand, maybe the analgesia we see in a fear situation has a different function, is just not the same as the analgesia or pain reduction you get when you're calming a patient with a placebo. If we try to think, not just mechanistically but organismically, we can begin to ask, well, why would we have evolved as animals that can do this, produce analgesia, and under what conditions does it make sense to do this? If you stick your hand into boiling water, that is not a good moment to produce an analgesic reaction. You want pain in that situation, because you want to know that you have to get that hand out immediately. On the other hand, if you are a soldier in combat and you get hit, it would be a very smart idea to give yourself a temporary shot of endogenous opiates or whatever it may be, just enough to get yourself off the battlefield, where it will then again be okay to feel the pain. So you begin to get the sense that analgesias may occur for different reasons under different kinds of circumstances, and that our discussion about the mechanisms involved needs to be framed within some kind of understanding of how they interact within a broader organismic motivational system.

Price: Well, I'm sure a number of people are thinking along those lines. Certainly, the refined analysis of what you are talking about begins to open up the distinction between fight or flight, between the battlefield situation where escape responses are made, and other circumstances where no escape is possible (like when you're lying in a hospital bed in severe pain). These kinds of concerns become very subtle and haven't been worked out. On the other hand, I wouldn't necessarily want to commit myself to making an a priori distinction between the analgesia of the battlefield and the analgesia you can get from a placebo in the clinic. Threat or fear translates into a clinical context as the thought, "I really want desperately to be relieved of pain"—and this has a powerful motivational effect.

Voodoo Death

Harrington: In this context, a phenomenon like voodoo death also seems to bring the question of where affect fits into these mind-body interactive processes right onto center stage. The original model of voodoo death, by Walter B. Cannon, supposed that it was not simply that you had an expectation of imminent death that then translated into the actual event. You were literally scared to death. There was a very strong affective load associated with the belief involved.

Barsky: There is a body of literature that's somewhat relevant to this question: the material on sudden cardiac death, which actually has been looked at fairly closely. It doesn't deal quite with the issue of expectation, but it does deal with the issue of the effect of intense emotion on a very measurable endpoint.

Reflecting on that literature, I think of two things that are sort of contrary. One of them is that a lot of the original work was done on pigs. And pigs are, I've been told, inordinately sensitive to stressful events, develop arrhythmias relatively easily, and can die suddenly.

But, on the other side, people have looked fairly carefully at the question of what precedes cases of sudden cardiac death, and quite often the extent of arousal and emotional stress doesn't appear to be all that powerful. It's rather hard to demonstrate that, for the most part, people who die suddenly do so immediately after some major and intense emotional experience.

Hyman: It is true, though, that when you study sleep, people do have more cardiac arrhythmias during REM sleep, when they are experiencing dreaming, than during other sleep stages.

Rose: Yes—the greatest incidence of myocardial infarctions occur early in the morning, after awaking from REM sleep.

Sullivan: There is literature on the Hmong, in Thailand and elsewhere, that speaks about a much higher incidence of people there dying during sleep and dreaming. For whatever reason, ethnographers have taken an interest in the kind of dream scenarios that seem to be associated with close calls or near-death experiences, where people can report. The results are very interesting, because the dreams identified with those experiences often culturally express certain notions of the dissolution of the self, and so on.

Benson: There are animal models for this. In a gruesome experiment a number of years ago, Richter took rather fierce wild rats and put them in Bell jars, half filled with water. The idea was to measure the amount of time they swam before they gave up and died. The mechanism of death was ventricular tachycardia, going on to ventricular fibrillation.

He found that the time was fairly consistent from onset of swimming to death. But then he altered the experiment. He took other, similar rats and put them in the jar, but before the expected time of death, he picked them up, held them a moment, and then put them back. And it turned out that the rats who experienced that brief reprieve swam much longer and lasted much longer than the rats who were left alone.

Now, we have problems attributing human emotions to rats, but could this not be pointing to something akin to hope of survival? There are other experiments which speak to the same phenomenon, in which hope is given in an otherwise hopeless situation. So I am wondering—and others have suggested this too—if voodoo death may not be fear, as much as it is hopelessness; and whether that is what is so deadly.

Stone: I think there is a lot to this point. I was once part of a group talking about dealing with dying patients; and there was a clinician there from the M. D. Anderson Clinic, who treated lots of children dying with cancer. He had developed a sort of semireligious, but I thought also empirical, thought about when to stop trying to treat the kid. He said, "You know, these kids can withstand a lot of pain, a lot of suffering. It is amazing how much pain a child can suffer. But when they lose hope, then you might as well give up on pushing more and more drugs."

Faith, Hope, and Healing

Price: So what is hope? When I first read papers on faith and hope, I had a hard time making sense of them because I was trying to translate the concepts into the psychological dimensions that we are more accustomed to dealing with as researchers. It finally occurred to me that hope has two factors implicit in it. Hope is where you have a desire *and* an expectation that are positive, going in the same direction. Faith may be a little more, a little different. But hope seems to have implicit in it, the notion of expectancy that Irving Kirsch is talking about, plus strong desire for something to happen. So, it seems to me that, if I'm right, then of course there is a general relationship between faith and hope and therapeutic effect.

Harrington: I wonder if there may be a way in which we need to understand hope as a structuring framework that allows you to withstand enormous amounts of pain because there is a larger context in which that pain is worth it and makes sense. I think of Alan Stone's story about the children with cancer, and then of Nietzsche's famous comment, that a person can hold out any "what," if he only has a "why." Seen from this view, hope would act as a motivational schema that isn't quite captured by concepts of "expectancy" and "desire."

Price: Well, expectancy and desire also constitute important variables for behavior and for motivation.

Harrington: I agree. I don't think it is a contradiction but I think it may be a spin of emphasis.

Brody: I was once very taken with a quotation I heard attributed to Vaclav Havel, who said that, "When we have hope, it doesn't mean that we think things will come out okay, it means that we think things will somehow make sense." So I think it is important to hold onto this idea that hope might be something more than just a passive emotion, it might involve a process by which people construct meaning to attach to events. And then we have to ask: why might there be something placebogenic about feeling that the things that are happening to you make sense? And where do we locate the active ingredient here? Does the "encounter" with a meaningful story of events set off certain psychosomatic pathways? Or is the active process of making your life meaningful, attaching meaning to events, somehow placebogenic?

Benson: I'm wondering about how to connect phenomena like hope to processes like meaning-making as well, and its healing effect. And I'm interested, in particular, in trying to relate both to religious behavior. On the one side, humans know they are mortal; it is this knowledge that perhaps differentiates us from other species. Knowing this, it is often very difficult for many to find meaning, especially when faced with a life-threatening illness. The meaning one might otherwise find in interpersonal relationships falls short because, again, you are dealing with another mortal.

So, one has to leave that framework to get the kind of meaning that then makes hopeful sense of life—a framework that for many involves belief in an afterworld. And so I wonder if we shouldn't start discussing meaningfulness and hope in terms of what seems to be a universal, almost hard-wired belief that there is "something beyond." Because it is just this kind of belief that often evokes what we would call the placebo effect, often through such practices as prayers and other religious behaviors.

Kaufman: Let me say something to underscore this point. When a religious believer says that he or she is placing all hope in the Lord, maker of heaven and earth, what is really being expressed is an assertion of where one draws one's deepest sense of security in the face of all the vicissitudes of life. There is a sense of resolve or commitment involved in deep hope of this sort, that is far more, I think, than simply a combination of expectancy and desire. It involves a process of admitting one's own inability to manage alone, and a willingness to lean back into some higher power—something that is far more than a combination of desire and expectation. It seems to me that this is the kind of deep hope that we should be particularly interested in, since it is this sort of hope that, we might imagine, enables healing to occur against the strongest odds, and in ways that seem very mysterious sometimes to modern medicine.

Harrington: I'm reflecting on how to connect what we are talking about here with our thinking about placebo effects as a more cognitive process—consequence of expectancy, as Irving Kirsch is urging us to do. It seems to me that expectancy has at least two dimensions: the formal state itself, and the content of that state. That is to say, you can imagine that there is something like a condition of *expectancy* in the abstract, but in fact there is always a specific content *to* expectancy. People expect *something*. This may seem obvious or trite, but it strikes me that actually the relationship between form and content here may not be so obvious. On the one side, you might imagine that there are degrees of intensity with which a person might expect something. You could kind of have an open mind, or you could be passionately, absolutely certain. Would you agree, Irving, that people who are really certain, really invested in their certainty, are probably going to have a more powerful immediate subjective, or physiological, response than those who are just kind of expecting something?

Kirsch: Yes, I think that's certainly right.

Harrington: But then, I was thinking: who are the most certain people? Maybe it's not those who have, in a sense, a very detailed map in their heads of what they imagine is going to happen, but rather the people who go to Lourdes and give themselves over to God and the mystery of healing. I had this idea that if a doctor gives you a very specific cognitive map of exactly how this dummy pill is going to work, then in a way he is disinvesting himself of just that kind of interpersonal charisma that allows him to function himself as such a powerful placebogenic agent. If you give a patient too much information, too much specificity, he or she may start to feel that this is just normal stuff after all. And in those cases, we might imagine that too much specificity undermines the capacity to have *faith,* or a kind of intense certainty that might be very placebogenic. So, somehow, there may be an interesting kind of tension between the necessity that an expectancy of healing be specific, and the necessity that the expectancy of healing be intense.

Kirsch: I agree with that entirely. And if you want to see that in operation, look at the work of skilled hypnotists, who will give suggestions like the following, during a hypnotic induction: "You may begin to notice, as you relax more and begin to enter hypnosis, you may begin to notice your hands beginning to tingle, or perhaps it will be your feet. And I wonder if you are more aware of your extremities becoming cold, or warm. You may sense a lightness in your left arm or a heaviness in your right arm. I wonder which you will be more aware of."

Consciousness and Conditioning

Hugdahl: Of course, a completely different, and much less mysterious, way to think about all these issues—one that is elegantly showcased in the work here of Bob Ader—is in terms of conditioning. But, even as the data is very compelling and the model is elegant, I also think there are enough anomalies in the total picture to push us to ask how well the traditional or classical view of placebo as a conditioned response—a simple, mechanical pairing of an active agent with a neutral one—how well that works when your sample is human, rather than animal? I was struck that Howard Fields spoke about a human conditioning group where, he said, previous experience of efficacy predicted the effect of the next placebo. This is a finding that is hard to reconcile with a classical conditioning view. And the key difference seems to me to involve a change in expectancy, or anticipation. The patient is anticipating something based on previous experience with something else. Yet, in classical conditioning, any process that involves changes in levels of anticipation or expectation should not make any differences to the outcome. So the standard view, in which automatic or reflexive behavior is elicited when a particular conditioned stimulus is presented, falls short. We need a more dynamic, top-down model of conditioning to explain placebo phenomenona, at least in humans.

Rose: Well, even in the animal model—and here I specifically take Bob Ader's work as an example—we could imagine that the conditioned response is dependent upon the animal's perception of the nature of the relationship between the placebo, the pairing of the saccharine to cyclophosphamide. If the animals were anesthetized and got it, you would not have gotten that effect.

Ader: That's right.

Rose: So what I think is interesting here is trying to figure out how, when you give the conditioned stimulus—in this case, the saccharine—it is having effects at the peripheral, cellular level similar to that produced by cyclophosphamide, that the learning can produce similar effects on the kidney and its basic membrane and its proteinuria as if the animals were getting the active drug.

We come back here to distinctions between illness and disease that we were struggling with before. Somehow you are not just affecting the animal's subjective state—the pain, the nausea, or whatever. You are actually affecting the peripheral biology; you are teaching the animal's body to mimic the effects of cyclophosphamide through the learned pairing to saccharine. So how can we understand that a learning process like this has this kind of powerful effect on the peripheral biology?

Ader: Of course I can't really answer your question. We do have some data which suggest that there may be some voluntary or instrumental behavioral components to explain part of this phenomenon, in the sense that animals with lupus will voluntarily consume solutions that contain cyclophosphamide in it to a greater extent than congenic controls. Now, how do they know that that is working? They have got to be able to perceive the change. This doesn't occur on Day One. If it occurred on Day One, I couldn't talk about learning. It takes them a week or two to figure it out and then they begin to drink more. Now, how do they know? Is that an immunologically derived signal to the nervous system, or is it an effect on the periphery? I can't answer your question yet. But I think it is an answerable question.

Jensen: Bob Ader said that if you anesthetized the animal during the time you were conditioning it, you wouldn't get this effect; do we know this to be true?

Ader: No, we don't know that to be true. You can certainly get conditioning without awareness, if you will; that is to say, without the subject being able to report exactly what is going on.

Jensen: It relates to this question of whether, if the subject knows that you are doing this conditioning, does it change the effect?

Ader: We have seen things like this with muscular sclerosis patients. There are some MS patients that are treated with cyclophosphamide, and we have looked at changes in white blood cell counts. We had ten subjects finish the whole protocol. They normally would get six active therapy sessions. I think they contracted for seven, and either the sixth or seventh was a sham, but it was either six *or* seven, so that the nurse also didn't know which was which.

Eight out of the ten patients showed a conditioned response in the white blood cell count; now, two of these didn't. One of those, we found out after the fact, had had a previous course of chemotherapy. This makes sense: preexposure to an unconditioned stimulus attenuates learning. The other patient recognized the conditioned stimulus as tasting like ouzo, with which he was familiar. This makes sense too: preexposure to the conditioned stimulus also attenuates learning. The two exceptions turned out to be strong support for the rule.

Now, the patients in general were also asked which trial they thought was the placebo. And one guy said, "I know which trial was the placebo." He was right, but it turned out he still showed the effect. Why? Because he could only figure it out after the fact. When you present the conditioned stimulus, a response is initiated. And afterwards he said, "Oh, I recognized . . ." But it was too late, he'd already responded. Now, next time around, in a long chemotherapy session, he is not going to know which one is real and which one isn't, so he is not going to be able to make that determination. In general, I think that foreknowledge may attenuate the response, but I do not think it will eliminate it.

Hyman: It seems like a pretty open question, what the role of the patient's subjectivity is likely to be in all of this, downstream of the initial eliciting effect. A lot of the circuitry that is probably engaged affectively, remains unconscious—processes having to do with the amygdala and the hypothalamus. There is actually a lot more going on in the brain, and a lot more going on in terms of outputs, than the subject is aware of.

Oepen: There are also cases that suggest things may be more complicated. Let me give you an example of a patient of mine that may be relevant to this point. He was schizophrenic, court-committed, and rather dangerous. I gave him haloperidol, and he got it by injection, so I knew it was in his system. Yet he did not respond well over five to six weeks and was really difficult to deal with. Every day I saw him and tried to explain to him why the treatment would be helpful for him, but he just remained very hostile.

After a while he said, "You know, doctor, you've been seeing me every day and have been polite to me and never really aggressive. So, I'm thinking—why don't I give this a chance, do it your way? I'll just take it—you don't have to give me the injections." I agreed, and what happened then was two things. First of all, he needed a much lower dose, because he was all of a sudden heavily sedated. He was being given high doses, a hundred milligrams of haloperidol a day, which hadn't done much to him before; but now he was really drowsy and also developed extrapyramidal side-effects.

The second thing that happened is that he had a notable benefit from the medication within a week. This is a much shorter time than it usually takes to see a benefit when you're just starting treatment, so the effect couldn't be explained by the onset of the oral medication. It was probably an accumulation of something that had been in the system before. Then he was able to tell me, "You know, I was fighting that drug the entire time you were injecting it. I was really hating you and the system and everything. I could feel the effect coming on and I was fighting it off, but it was difficult. The moment I agreed to take the drug, though, I let it take over, just let myself give in." A situation much like Gordon Kaufman was speaking of before. And that was when he had both the benefits and the side-effects and needed a much lower dose.

Meaning-Making, Psychotherapy, and the Power of Stories

Brody: You know, we can emphasize the passivity of these processes, letting go and so on, but I remain attached to a more active model that focuses on the placebogenic properties of what I call meaning-making. And I believe strongly that the making of meaning happens through the construction of narratives, the creation and telling of stories. The psychologist Jerome Bruner makes a great deal of this point: according to Bruner, stories or narratives are the main way we have of making sense of events around us. And what is a narrative? Basically, it is a way of situating ourselves in relation to an experience, in relation to other important people, for a specified period of time. It is key to understanding a narrative to see that it has a beginning, a middle, and an ending. And so that is a way of creating a structured, finite model of ourselves in the world, that allow us to attach meaning to events by locating the relationships between event A, event B, and so in a temporal sequence, in a kind of quasi-causal way—what happens first, what happens next? In this way, narratives give us *back* active control, give us reason to assume we can predict events occurring, and this may be placebogenic.

Harrington: So you are saying, Howard Brody, that healing happens when we tell a story that allows us to make sense of our situation. I find this fascinating, because one of the big concerns people have had about trying to do controlled studies of psychotherapy is that it appears that there is no placebo you can introduce, because in a sense, all psychotherapy is a placebo. That is, there are words and interactions.

But what you just taught me, or what I began to think as you were talking, is that effective psychotherapy may involve more than just any old mix of words and interactions. Effective psychotherapy provides both patient and psychotherapist with a systematized story in which both can immerse themselves and set those placebogenic processes you were talking about, into play. That means that psychoanalysis, for example, might be completely wrong, according to external, scientific standards. But it nevertheless might work very effectively if both patient and psychoanalyst are committed to the story it tells about human beings. In fact, the most true story that something like science may be able to develop of human behavior at the same time may not be the most subjectively persuasive story for either patient or therapist; that is, in your terms, the most placebogenic story.

Brody: George Engel made an interesting comment in one of his essays about the fascinating parallelism of processes in the doctor/patient relationship. What allows doctors and patients to relate and communicate so readily, as strangers, in a time of great crisis? Engel felt that there are needs, almost biologically driven in nature, that are complementary. The doctor has this biologically driven need to understand, and the patient has a biologically driven need to be understood.

Sullivan: Another way to consider what we are talking about here is by asking how narratives participate in the symbolic constitution of the person. People are made up of more than just their material stuff; they are literally products of their culture's symbols too. And here I am particularly interested in Howard Brody's discussion of how, in the psychotherapeutic setting, a person's life experience is suddenly shoehorned into a psychoanalytic narrative, let's say. Well, that isn't the life itself, that's a map of the territory of one's experience. But you manipulate the map to change the territory, so to speak. Here I am thinking of the philosopher, Paul Ricoeur, who looked at the psychoanalytic narrative, really as a way of manipulating time. If a person's existence in time can be cast into symbolic form, into a narrative, especially a psychoanalytic narrative, then one can manipulate the model of the person's life in that ritual setting; experience is poured into symbolic forms, so to speak, and made manipulable. The fact that manipulation happens inside a ritual space is also key to seeing how this can work: I wrote down here a quote from Jonathan Smith that, "ritual represents the creation of a controlled environment, where the variables and accidents of ordinary life may be displaced, precisely because they are felt to be so overwhelmingly present and powerful." So, in psychotherapy, as I understand it, the accidents and stuff of real life that are overwhelming the patient can be displaced. A kind of clearing is being made.

Hyman: Right—through the formation of organizing narratives, for example. Which is a lot of what, previously, I heard people calling placebo.

Brody: And the point here is that *both* the doctor and the patient are symbiotically involved in the process, with healing being the ultimate goal. So, this points to a fascinating picture of the symbiotic nature of the doctor/patient relationship, and the ways in which this relationship creates a process somehow stimulatory of the psychosomatic pathways.

Rose: It's like Arthur Kleinman says: making meaning is many heads; it's not just one head doing it.

Culture in the Body

Kosslyn: Let's see if we can fit this into the observations we've made so far. Not long ago, I got an infected kidney and was really laid up incredibly badly. It incapacitated me completely for five days. The striking thing was that it waited to strike until Thanksgiving, when I had a lot of time for vacation and had no work that was due. It was amazing.

That was not the first time something like this had happened to me. In fact, once Anne Harrington noticed that I waited until vacations to get sick, and she said, "you shouldn't let yourself get sick." And I thought, "I'm not responsible." Then I thought, "Well, gee, what a coincidence." So, I'm wondering whether there is something to this, being able to use a social hook to hold a disease process back and then at some point you get overwhelmed.

Spiro: I'll just interrupt you to say that it is an interesting metaphor to use in relation to kidney trouble.

Kosslyn: I was going to get to that. I've been told that it is much more common for old people to die during the week following their birthday than the week immediately before their birthday. And there was a study that showed that traditional Chinese are less likely to die during Chinese holidays than during Jewish ones, and vice versa for Orthodox Jews.

It is clear that Thanksgiving, in my case, and things like birthdays and holidays in general, are cultural constructs. How is it that a factor like that can influence our bodies? How does Thanksgiving influence my body? Aside from the obvious, gluttony way.

Sullivan: I am quite interested, and yet not very surprised, that significant days in the calendar year can mix themselves into people's constitutions that way. I started talking about this before, when we were talking about how narratives may function in psychotherapy, but let me take it up again. I don't know how many people keep a day book or something, but scholars who have studied the phenomenology of time consciousness have shown how people's whole experiential lives are shaped by the calendar. Time, special dates, become constituent parts of their consciousness, and are intertwined with the setting of goals for themselves, having relationships, and so on. We all have these kinds of controlling temporal devices built into our constitutions.

Harrington: So, going back to Steve Kosslyn's questions, even something as apparently ephemeral as time can end up being symbolically rendered in all sorts of artifacts in our world—our day books, our calendars. And I think you're suggesting, Larry, that our engagement with these artifacts may actually evoke meaningful changes in our physiological processes?

Sullivan: Yes, and it seems to me that these kinds of representations of temporal structures may be present and available for triggering even in some of the objects whose effects we otherwise are prone to explain in mechanistic, causal ways, such as active medications. There are clear notions about time that are packed into processing of synthetic drugs, designed to imitate what occurs naturally over a longer time course. The more general point here is that there is a dense condensation of our cultural symbols even inside objects that appear to us culturally inert, so to speak.

Kleinman: On this larger question of what Larry Sullivan is alluding to—what we can call sociosemantic transformation—I think there are a number of very interesting mediators, even beyond time and narrative, where our attention could and should be given. One turns on the way that the moral engages the affective: the embodiment of the moral. The Chinese have a very simple way of talking about this, they call it Lianzani Face. Face is both a dimension of social experience, referring to your moral worth in the community, but it is also literally your embodiment of culture. When you figuratively lose face, when you're humiliated, as people were in the Cultural Revolution, you also literally lose face, physically the face crumbles downward. This suggests that moral belief is not just an idea, but is deeply affective. It's not a convention you can take on and take off like at an academic roundtable.

Sullivan: And, in terms of our interdisciplinary dialogue, it does go some way toward undermining the notion that when you're trying to fit together the neurobiology and the sociocultural dimensions of this phenomenon, only grave topics are going to float to the bottom of the ladder of levels, to the neurobiological foundations, while all topics that are perceived as being somehow lighter than air stay up there in the sociocultural world.

Kleinman: On this point, one great challenge, as I see it, to doing this kind of work right, lies in removing obstacles to the way we think about placebos and other mind/body processes; obstacles that come from the ideological biases of western science itself. As a medical anthropologist, I will tell you that one of the most profound things about western biomedicine that differentiates it from every other system of medicine we know of in the world—as well as from western medicine prior to about the end of the seventeenth century— is its antivitalism. Its antivitalism, which we take as one of its chief achievements, is in fact what differentiates it from all other forms of healing.

If you look at other theories of healing, much of what they would regard as the central mediators between the social and the physiological, the interpersonal and the personal, are indeed things like power, vital energy, movement, *qi*. In Chinese medicine, *qi* literally means "movement," it means "power." I would suggest that there must be a way in which, from a neurobiological standpoint, cognitive neuroscience and neurobiology might want to configure that phenomenological observation of energy and power in treatment. Whether you conceive of it as "charisma," or whether you see it in some other transformative way, its absence as an explanatory construct in biomedicine restricts potential for deeper understanding.

Stigmas and Physician Anxieties

Spiro: I am impressed by the fact that there is very little discussion of placebos in medical institutions, just as there is very little discussion of death in medical institutions. We are ashamed of death; it is a kind of defeat for us. Similarly, there is something shameful about using a placebo. We are taught at Harvard Medical School, Yale Medical School, and other places to be scientists. We are taught to use things that will work logically, empirically, et cetera, et cetera. The placebo reminds us that we still have cousins out there who are witch doctors, who are shamans, who are all kinds of things. And doctors just don't like to admit that kind of thing.

Sullivan: Let me just say to that, popular scientific opinion to the contrary, no self-respecting shaman or magical healer that I have ever met would want to describe the core of his or her practice as placebo either. And although we've pointed out that the term "placebo" is drawn from a Catholic liturgical context, no religion would want to identify its healing system as placebo therapy either. So biomedical practice is no different than any of these other systems, even though there seems to be widespread consensus that placebo processes are widely operative at many levels of general practice.

Kleinman: Yet one would think that we would want to educate our students in such a way as to assure the maximum kind of placebo response that we're producing anyway routinely in care. Yet, by and large, we seem to look at the placebo response as a kind of a dirty contaminant in the research process.

Now why is this? I think it must be because it gets at certain dimensions of human functions that we don't know much about and that are threatening in some way to medicine. And, so we don't build on it in our training so we don't have to confront the larger implication of the phenomenon.

Hyman: You know, in psychiatry it's very striking. There is a generation of psychopharmacologists who basically see honest real treatment as involving a process in which this pill interacts with this receptor. As cleanly as possible, they divorce themselves from psychotherapeutic approaches in the field, which they treat, not as science, but as art, which is to say, practically fraud or shamanism. They really want very strongly to believe that the only thing that occurs when you treat depression with, say imipramine or Prozac, is an interaction between a chemical and a receptor. Yet, to challenge the sufficiency of that view is not necessarily to challenge the adequacy of the biomedical frame in general, as I think Arthur Kleinman was suggesting. I think, rather, that we have to take it as a good hypothesis that the brain is very susceptible, not only to these specific pharmacologic locks and keys, but to contextual variables besides. Moreover, not all systems in the brain are equally susceptible to alteration of contextual variables. Systems dealing with pain and affective states may be much more responsive to interpersonal and contextual variables than, say, systems that produce a brain tumor, which may be why we tend to focus on apparently more stable phenomena like that. But in fact, I would think the whole point of having a mammalian brain is to be able to adapt and to be able to learn, and that means being highly sensitive to signals and information from the context.

In this sense, part of the reason for placebo's negative image, for the ways in which biomedicine dismisses the importance of physician-patient relationship and the power of narrative, is that most people are bad neurobiologists and think, if I can't explain the phenomenon using a rigid, lock-key algorithm, then it's nothing but mystical hokum.

So to admit a role for interpersonal and contextual variables in healing is not to admit that you believe in magic; there really is a neurobiology here that we should be able to study, that engages neural circuitry and so on. To think about the mechanisms involved in these variables is not only to target an interesting research domain—I think more research of this sort may also liberate physicians in the clinic to embrace these kinds of factors much more wholeheartedly, to stop being ashamed of them, and indeed try to maximize their efficacy.

Scarry: I agree. There is something odd about the fact that much of what we are hearing described, in terms of the actual outcome of placebo effect, is by most people's account, extremely positive. And yet, we keep then falling back into the very negative connotations of the word "placebo effect," a word that seems to imply trickery and sham. The discrepancy is actually quite startling.

I believe fully that no one, from physicians to psychoanalysts to shamans, would want to have the negative connotations we attach to the placebo effect attributed to their practices. But certainly they would want to have attributed to them the very positive outcomes we have heard described. So how can we preserve the sense of the latter, while distancing ourselves from the negative ideas of trickery and sham, which are discrediting both to the patient and to the physician?

Howard Spiro suggested an alternative vocabulary: instead of placebo, call it the seal on the contract between physician and patient; a sign of the physician's commitment to healing his or her patient. Other vocabularies suggest themselves. For example, the notion of thinking of either the physician or the pill as a kind of lens through which the amorphous contextual and interpersonal thing we have been talking about is somehow going to get focused and brought to bear on the emergency of the sickness, whatever it is. Those symbolic processes are supposedly operating all the time, and yet, in a situation of illness or disease, there is a special need to try to focus and concentrate those resources on the specific problem. So, "lens" might be another word.

In general, it might be useful if people consciously reflect on the phrases in which they are thinking of placebo, and actually offer the vocabulary up to us. Because otherwise we are likely to keep rein-heriting all the connotations of trickery and sham. And we can't afford to, because the highest aspirations of the medical profession are at stake in some of these outcomes.

Deception, Autonomy, and the Ethics of Placebo Use

Stone: There is a standard parable in medical ethics that deals with our subject that I've been teaching for fifteen years; so I've had a chance to listen to 1500 law students discuss it, as well as doctors. A Mr. Marks is admitted into the hospital with respiratory decompensations. He's had respiratory problems for many years. When he comes in now, they have to decide whether they're going to put him on a respirator or not. They don't really want to put him on the respirator, but he's having enough trouble that they put him in the intensive care unit. And he keeps complaining to the doctor, "Doctor, Doctor, I'm in pain, I want something for my pain."

And the doctor, either rightly or wrongly, concludes that if he gives him something for pain, it will compromise his breathing. So he tells the nurse, "Give him a cc of saline." So, they inject Mr. Marks with a cc of saline, and he quietly goes to sleep. The nurses are relieved. The doctor is relieved. But the question is: was this ethical?

Now, the reason it might not be ethical is, as you all clearly understand, that we have this notion that people are supposed to have choice. They're supposed to have autonomy about their medical treatment. The upshot of the whole evolution of the concept of informed consent is the insistence that doctors tell you what they're doing to you before they do it, so you can choose whether you want it or not.

Now, there's some sense in which we around this table would probably wonder whether you can get a placebo response in a situation of absolute informed consent. Yet that's what the law requires. So, this doctor knows, when he gives this injection, that he's done something that, according to contemporary standards of ethics and law, is not quite right. Even though it produces a benefit. Even though it provides the patient with the least pathological treatment that accomplishes the same good. The thing is, we live in an age in which, from a legal point of view and a moral point of view, autonomy trumps everything else.

Spiro: Back in the 1940s, when I was at Harvard Medical School, there were catalogs of pills that you could buy cheaply. And in that catalog, there also were several pages of placebos. They came in blue and yellow and green and all the rest, and doctors were perfectly happy to have them. But then, in the 1960s, as you say, we saw the beginnings of the autonomy movement, along with the derogation of paternalism, now called parentalism, as hierarchically disparate. This all sort of destroyed the notion that doctors could comfortably use placebos. But of course, in fact, we still do. We use them all the time. We use them in diagnostic studies, we use them in operations, we use them even in my field of gastroenterology.

Scarry: Would there be the same ethical dilemma if the physician were to put the situation to Mr. Marks in the way that Howard Spiro told us he puts matters to his patients? Presumably the physician could say, "I have a choice in prescribing medication for your pain. I can either give you a substance which will interfere with your breathing, and the advantage is I understand how this substance works. Or, I can give you another substance that I know will not interfere with your breathing and that I have reason to believe will work equally well, but I don't, myself, understand how it works."

Stone: If he does that with a patient, there's no problem. But now let's say he wants to get a grant and do research, and he says, "I want to use that language, which I use all the time with my patients, in my protocol." If he wants to get funded, then it's going to have to go to the human rights committee, and somebody is going to begin to raise questions whether there is, in this, something of a deception.

Scarry: But only because we've so associated sham and trickery with placebo. In fact, if it's going to have that outcome, then there is no trick.

Stone: I quite agree with you. It doesn't have to be that way. If the doctor believed that saline was an effective pain analgesic, then there would be no deception.

Kirsch: You said that there may not be as great a problem for the physician with an individual patient as there would be for the researcher confronted with an institutional review board. Just two points about that. One is that deception is, under certain circumstances, allowed as an ethical research procedure, though it requires debriefing and some justification. Second, and more specific to the question of placebo and placebo research, there's a very elegant research design that allows us to get around some of the pitfalls of the informed consent combined with double-blind design, and that's the balanced placebo design.

The way in which that typically works is as follows. The informed consent initially is the same as it would normally be, "You're going to be in an experiment, some of the people in the experiment are going to get an active drug, some are going to be in a control group and not get it." Then the person is informed, "You are getting the active drug, or you are in the control group and are not getting the active drug." For half the people that information is true, for half the people, that information is deceptive.

This design gives you a very nicely balanced set of four cells in which people are either (1) knowingly getting the drug; (2) getting the placebo and being informed that they're getting a drug; (3) getting a drug but thinking they're not getting it; or, (4) not getting a drug and knowing they're not getting a drug. This design has many, many advantages over typical double-blind designs, and it's produced tremendous information. At the end, as in double-blind studies, the subjects are debriefed.

Spiro: In the everyday world of the clinic, more and more I detect a growing recognition that doctors are specialists licensed by the state, and that we therefore do have a right, if not a duty, to be somewhat more authoritarian than the past thirty years has permitted us to be. In a sense, I see things moving back to the middle. People are talking about virtue again. They are talking about beneficence. I think there is a swing of the pendulum.

Brody: I think you're absolutely right to stress that the current concept of autonomy is predominantly a legalistic concept of autonomy, and agree that it's terribly inadequate. But what I hope will happen is not that the pendulum will swing back to the middle, but the next logical advance will take us beyond our current limited notion of autonomy so that we will understand that as individuals we are, in fact, socioculturally embedded and not the Marlboro Man. That is to say, our relationships with others and our dependency upon others is part of our selfhood. This richer concept of autonomy could, I think, very strongly promote acceptance of the placebo response in clinical care.

What am I going to say to this new kind of autonomous patient? Certainly, I'm not going to deceive him. For me to deceive my patients feels like something similar to my poisoning the ecosystem. I won't contaminate the system that way. So what I'm going to say to my autonomous patient is, "I want to be trustworthy. I think trust is a pivotal aspect of the doctor-patient relationship and good healing. If I want you to trust me, I have to be trustworthy. Therefore, I want to be sure that I tell you the truth. I don't want to engage in a relationship with you where you wonder periodically am I deceiving you or withholding information. So, my job is to be trustworthy. Now let me tell you some new findings that have highlighted for us all the mechanisms you have built into your own brain and your own body and that allow you, when you are in the right frame of mind, when you trust, when you have the right therapeutic milieu, to contribute tremendously to the potency of whatever pill I may give you. So you, as an autonomous being, have tremendous power within yourself to heal yourself. So let us work together in a trusting, mutual relationship in which I can contribute something to your healing and you can contribute something to your healing." Now, that is moving into a whole new direction. It's not a pendulum swing back to the authoritarian position, but rather something that moves us towards a much richer concept of autonomy.

Spiro: A secondhand car salesman says, "Trust me." In the real world in which we live, patients are not really able to take in all that information, or feel responsible for their own healing. We're talking about the "ideal patient" the way the lawyers talk about the "prudent person," or economists talk about the "economic man." In the real world—at least the world that I've dealt with—patients are sick, they want help, they are not in a position, really, to say, "Well, let me think about all of this for a time." They say, "Doctor, what do *you* think I should do?" They don't need and they don't want to be full, responsible partners.

Somebody earlier in our conversation said, "Well, giving up control is the first step towards healing." And you know, the stories we have collected on sick doctors, it was perfectly clear that when doctors gave up and said, "Take care of me," they felt much better, and they did much better.

Brody: What I see in my patients is a situation where doctors and patients stay together over time, do learn how to get along, do learn how to trust, do learn rapport, and do invest in a relationship. Now, that's a family practice model at a Midwestern university instead of a gastroenterology model at Yale. And, of course, your model is the more typical model. Your model is the dominant model in American medicine, and there's a lot of argument as to how far that kind of model plays into why American medicine is in trouble socioeconomically. In this sense, we need to talk about how, if you're going to make placebo a more central part of medicine, then somehow in the process you are going to have to reform medical thinking across the board. You can't really define placebo and not challenge the biomedical model and the dominant thought patterns, including some of the socioeconomic assumptions, that support it.

Stone: Howard Brody, your view of the doctor-patient relationship—which I think many of us around this table would espouse—is being transformed by managed care in such a way that it's going to be increasingly difficult for patients, at least in urban areas, to hope for such a relationship. Now, given that, poised where we are in socioeconomic and historical time, do we want to say, "Okay doctors, use placebos?" There is this problem of what happens when placebos are taken out of the benevolent doctor's hands. Doctors will give patients injections of antibiotics, just because they'll go away happy. They'll say that *Kaiser Permanente* is good health care because they got what they wanted.

Spiro: One of the scenarios with which I challenge medical students and residents goes as follows: You're in the ER; the patient has a ruptured liver. He's on his way to the operating room. You walk in; his wife is holding his hand. The orderly is wheeling the patient out towards the operating room, and the patient looks up at you and says, "Doc, am I going to make it?"

And you know what? Most of the time the residents and other doctors trained in the past ten to fifteen years will give a weasel answer, "Well, maybe, we're going to try." Nobody is willing anymore to grab that patient's hand and give the reassurance, "*Sure* you're going to make it." They give two reasons. One is, "I want to tell the truth, I've been raised to tell the truth, I don't believe he's going to make it, I shouldn't tell him that he's going to make it if I don't think he is." And the other one is, of course, the malpractice issue, which I point out to them is easily handled—you take the wife aside and explain what you think.

Stone: You see, all these things make sense to us because we have a certain level of faith in the reality of caring doctors, but that kind of faith is foreign to people who are concerned about autonomous choice, people who want to make patients equal bargaining partners in a contractual relationship. But it's not yet clear at what cost to the more elusive aspects of the doctor-patient relationship that we've been discussing around the table today.

The Future of Placebo Research and the Challenge of Interdisciplinarity

Sullivan: I think one lesson I'm learning from these conversations is that every topic we propose comes from somewhere. There's no view from nowhere. If you toss the topic up from one of the various domains that claim it, gravity eventually overcomes the issue, and it does return to Earth somewhere in the vicinity of where it went up. For me, this means that the process of choosing topics matters; that a certain self-consciousness about the implications of setting the problem up this way or that way will be important. For example, we've talked about pain as a paradigm for placebo effects, but this was pain as self-presented in the clinic. Our discussions would have been very different if we took our starting point from something like Elaine Scarry's book on pain; that is, the comparative literature of pain on the one hand and political torture on the other. So we are really going to need to cash out the implications of our different choices, and see which are going to act as the most fruitful structure and prod for interdisciplinary conversation.

Brandt: It seems to me that when one thinks about what the goals of an interdisciplinary dialogue on placebo might be, perhaps we should actually be wary of taking for granted that a grand theory that combines the best of everyone's world should be our goal. Perhaps, instead, placebo can serve us as a kind of entry point for a number of different disciplines talking a lot to one another in ways that may reshape the way they conceptualize problems in their own field. Rather than looking for a common theoretical umbrella to unite us, we may seek other kinds of strategies to bring us together: it seems to me, for example, that we might identify the clinic as a common site in which complex processes occur that could benefit from the perspectives of multiple disciplines. So a site of action becomes an opportunity for cross-disciplinary dialogue in which the different partners maintain their intellectual heterogeneity even while seeking to learn from one another.

Kaufman: To a certain extent, I must confess that I'm less optimistic about what the outcome of such conversations might be than perhaps many of you. As far as I can see, the concept of placebo at its core is a kind of negative artifact of the enormous growth of our medical knowledge over the past couple of centuries. I've been quite struck about the extent to which placebo seems to signify ignorance to a great many medical people. It is the place, you might say, in modern medicine where a kind of awareness comes into focus that there is a great deal about human healing and human disease that we really don't understand. Placebo is the place where modern medical knowledge confronts its limits, confronts what theologians call human finititude, to use a big word. We humans have a great deal of power. We have knowledge that enables us to do all kinds of very amazing things. But there are limits. In this respect, the placebo phenomenon directs us toward some of the very large questions about human life: the limitations of our knowledge and what kind of meaning life can have in the face of that. We haven't pursued these issues very much here. These are questions that the great religious traditions have always spoken about and might have some wisdom to offer to us.

Brandt: Well, in a somewhat less exalted sense, I agree that placebo does function as a definition about limits. Defining the placebo effect is a question at the core of how medicine works, or what it means to say that medicine works in the first place. As a medical historian, it's always been my conviction that medicine has always "worked." On the other hand, some people would say, "But medicine, until the most recent periods, has been merely a 'placebo effect.'" So our definition of that term—and how we judge the phenomenon it describes—captures a lot of tensions about how we construe effective, good medicine in our time.

Biomedicine and the social sciences are likely to come up with different kinds of definitions or models of the placebo effect, not only because biomedicine is what some people call reductionistic, and the social sciences focus more on context, but also because they have different goals in terms of what they want to know. One of the primary goals of biomedicine and bioscience is to come up with universalizing views of the body and universalizing generalizations that say, "with a given doctor and a given patient, we can elicit these kinds of generalizable, predictable effects." And one of the characteristics of a certain kind of thinking within the social and cultural sciences is an emphasis on differentiation and distinction; the insistence on not making generalizations beyond the local, immediate situation.

Hyman: But the real issue is, when do each of us say, "Now I understand?" Now, an extreme reductionist never really understands anything, right? I mean, if I were to draw a map of the electron probability waves in our brains, I would certainly never understand the emergent properties of something like a placebo. So I think we can forget about very naive reductionism. Yet, I still have a feeling that, while I accept, for example, that interpersonal interactions, the doctor-patient relationship, and so on are privileged stimuli in placebo processes, I want to know *why* they are privileged from the point of view of the brain. For *me* to feel that I understand, I need to know a mechanism. I need to know that something like a caring encounter with a physician is going to alter synaptic weights and have, therefore, certain implications for subsequent experience and for behavioral outputs. And I suspect that other people would feel differently; they wouldn't say, "Now I understand," if they got an explanation in that form.

Scarry: Steve Hyman said, if I understood him correctly, that he would feel that he had reached some kind of resting point when he had a neurobiological model of placebo action, but he assumed that other people might feel differently about that.

What I want to say is that, I don't see how that could not be an outcome we would *all* want. I realize that some of us want to emphasize a more intermediate space that concentrates on bridging elements; and, since I work in literature and with theories of narrative, of course I'm committed to that perspective. At the same time, I can't understand how a neurobiological model could not be the most desirable outcome for everyone. While it's important not to forget that the processes through which one arrives at knowledge about the brain are often very reductionist, the brain mechanisms themselves are not reductionist. The brain mechanisms themselves are as extraordinary and as exhilarating as any poem by Yeats.

Harrington: But the brain is not itself alone. The brain is also a symbol of the authority of one discipline over another discipline, of the privileging of one language over another—it is, as Larry Sullivan reminded us before, a "view from somewhere." In that sense, how can we insure that the brain model of placebo we come up with exists in a realm where it is an interdisciplinary object rather than an object for which only one discipline has defined the language and epistemological standards?

Scarry: Well, we know that there already exist biological models that can accommodate social and cultural factors in quite supple ways, such as the Gate Control Theory of Pain. One may or may not accept that particular theory, but it's an example of where a future interdisciplinary approach to placebo action might develop. No model that fails to account for the interpersonal and contextual factors we've been describing today could possibly be accurate; but that's just the first reason we need to be sure we build them into future neurobiological theories.

Oepen: Elaine, I would like to give an example which may help to make it more clear why I think your way of thinking is dangerous, even while it's very appealing.

If you make a Fourier analysis of a musical piece, this is a great method to analyze sound, and it gives you true, excellent data. But those data have nothing to do with music, even though you can analyze the harp and the violin or the trombone and do other fancy things. But in a sense, you've still missed the point, because that's not music.

Scarry: But you're taking what is an unacceptable or not-yet satisfactory model of the brain; a model, for example, in which all it's being asked to do is to account for its reaction to this chemical or that inhibiting chemical. That kind of approach doesn't yet accommodate the things that the placebo research would demand of the brain—that it explain how it comes to respond to the voice or touch of a concerned physician, to an impressive injection procedure, and so on.

Moreover, once one had a model like that, it wouldn't be a way of displacing the music. It's not as though you throw out the harp and the violin once you understand something about how the brain hears the music. You don't throw out colors once you have an account of how color vision works. It doesn't mean you stop seeing colors.

Hyman: Godehard, I also think you've made it too easy for yourself. Nobody thinks that a Fourier transform is a good explanation for the enjoyment of music. You have to make it harder for yourself and ask what kind of understanding would you have if you looked at the interactions between the music that is perceived, as decoded by the auditory mechanisms, the symbolic outputs that are then produced, and the limbic mechanisms that give the emotional color to the judgment of those outputs. If you knew all that, would you admit that you knew something about the neurobiology of music?

I think we really have to butt heads not with the straw man reductionists who really explain nothing, but with the real question of at what point you are going to be able to say, "Now I understand why music is beautiful to me."

Kosslyn: The ideology, if I can call it that, of cognitive neuroscience—my own discipline—is something called nonreductionist materialism. The idea is that you can't replace—eliminate—talk of mental activities like memory perception, mental imagery, and so on, by talk of the brain. But we believe that these mental phenomena arise through a complex set of interactions at the level of the brain. This leads to the realization that, depending on the question you ask, different things count as answers. It's not as if there's a competition between different levels of description, because they're complementary.

Ader: What we need here is somebody who will defend what you're calling the reductionistic biomedical model; not somebody who is going to agree with the guy sitting next to him all the time, but someone who's going to say, "Prove it, show me, don't tell me about it. Why should I accept the position you are taking with respect to these phenomena?" You need a foil like this, but a good one, someone who is really good.

Kleinman: Well, I wanted to respond to Elaine Scarry's comments. I agree that it would be impossible to conceive an outcome for an interdisciplinary examination of placebo effects that did not include an extraordinarily important input from neurobiology. But I would say at the same time that, for the outcome to be as robust as one would want it to be, then you've got to come to terms in a complex and sophisticated way with the social world. We must be careful not to allow a kind of discreetness and rigor to prevail in our neurobiological thinking without matching it on the other side. Because, believe me, there is also a rigor to the way that metaphors move through social space, the way that rituals become part of the cultural body in the phenomenology of lived experience. The culturalist program needs to be very detailed and very specific. Of course it has to engage the specificity of the neurologic and neurobiological program, but it shouldn't be forced to do that too early.

Scarry: On one level, I agree with you, of course. And, on another level, I really don't agree with you, and I want to try to say why. I start by describing my own experience that I suspect will resonate also with you and many other people in this room. As humanists, you go around to the medical schools, and you speak to scientists, and so forth. By giving persuasive, rigorous accounts of the way metaphor works and the way narrative works, occasionally a tiny number of people become convinced that one can't practice or study medicine without taking those things into account.

I refer to this as a small number of conversions. And even here, the fact that I was invited to speak meant that the people to whom I was speaking, the people who invited me, were open to my views, were ready to be converted. What, though, if you could go to all the rest of the people, who would never think to go to a talk on metaphor and narrative and say, "Look, there's been a kind of breakthrough in neurobiological thinking that makes clear that sociocultural factors are not just a postscript to certain physical processes that happen in the body; in fact, they're active right at the front door."

Howard Spiro has remarked that probably all of us at this table wish our physicians would listen to us more. Now that's a remarkable thought. On the one hand, it's widely known that everyone wishes that; but on the other hand, it doesn't just come about. Until these things have been conceptualized in terms of their "real" demands on the brain and the body, medical practice just isn't going to take them seriously. It's true that everyone *here* is already committed to a dialogue between the sciences and the humanities—otherwise we wouldn't be here—but this kind of openness is not descriptive of the medical industry at large. So I believe strongly that humanistic changes in medical practice will only come once they're justified in terms of the principles of biomedical science and neuroscience.

Kosslyn: Elaine, I agree, but I think you're misnaming the end point. By the time we've reached a model that truly can account for all the things you're asking of it, then it no longer is "just" a neurobiological model; it's something more than that. It's something that integrates, that blurs what we consider to be the self "inside" and the self "outside." And when a way of thinking like that is established, we won't be just doing neurobiology. We will be doing something new, something integrative that we can't yet fully imagine.

Contributors
Index

Contributors

Robert Ader received his Ph.D. in experimental psychology from Cornell University in 1957. Currently, he is the George L. Engel Professor of Psychosocial Medicine and Director of the Division of Behavioral and Psychosocial Medicine in the Department of Psychiatry at the University of Rochester School of Medicine and Dentistry. He is also the Director of an Interdepartmental Center for Psychoneuroimmunology Research in the School of Medicine and Dentistry. In addition, Dr. Ader is the editor of *Psychoneuroimmunology* (1981), coeditor of the Second Edition of that work (1991), and editor-in-chief of the journal *Brain, Behavior, and Immunity*.

Howard Brody received his M.D. and Ph.D. (Philosophy) from Michigan State University and completed a residency in Family Practice at the University of Virginia. He is Professor of Family Practice and Philosophy and directs the Center for Ethics and Humanities in the Life Sciences at Michigan State University. The author of *Placebos and the Philosophy of Medicine* (University of Chicago Press, 1980), he is interested in the philosophical and ethical aspects of the placebo effect and the role of the placebo response in the physician-patient relationship in primary care medicine.

Howard L. Fields is a neurologist and nuerobiologist who is Professor of Neurology and Physiology at the University of California, San Francisco. He received his M.D. and Ph.D. in Neuroscience from Stanford University and trained in Neurology at Harvard Medical School. He has made major contributions to our understanding of the physiology and pharmacology of pain and its control.

Robert A. Hahn received his Ph.D. in anthropology at Harvard University in 1976 and his M.P.H. in epidemiology from the University of Washington in 1986. Since 1986, he has served as an epidemiologist at the U.S. Centers for

Disease Control and Prevention in Atlanta. Also, he has conducted anthropological and public health research in Peru, Mexico, Brazil, the United States, Niger, and the Cameroon. He has published studies on a variety of topics, including breast cancer and other chronic diseases, syphilis, AIDS, obstetrics, internal medicine in the United States, perinatal ethics, race and ethnicity as categories in public health, poverty, death, and male-female differences in mortality. Dr. Hahn is the author of *Sickness and Healing: An Anthropological Perspective* (Yale, 1995). "The Nocebo Phenomenon: Scope and Foundations" was prepared by the contributor as part of official duties as an employee of the Federal Government/Centers for Disease Control and Prevention. The copyright in *The Placebo Effect* does not extend to this chapter.

Anne Harrington is Professor in the History of Science at Harvard University, specializing in the history of psychiatry, neuroscience, and other mind sciences. She received her Ph.D. in the History of Science from Oxford University in 1985. Currently she is a consultant for the MacArthur Foundation Research Network on Mind-Body Interactions. She is also co-director of the Harvard University Mind, Brain, Behavior Initiative. In addition to writing over forty articles and producing two edited collections, she is author of two books, *Mind, Medicine, and the Double Brain* (1987) and *Reenchanted Science: Holism and German Culture from 1890–1945* (Princeton University Press, 1996).

Irving Kirsch is a Professor of Psychology at the University of Connecticut. He is a former president of the American Psychological Association's Division of Psychological Hypnosis and the current North American Editor of the international journal, *Contemporary Hypnosis*. Dr. Kirsch is an author or editor of five books and more than one hundred journal articles and book chapters.

David Morris is the author of numerous scholarly essays and three award-winning books, including *The Culture of Pain* (1991), which received a prestigious PEN prize. A recent book of his is *Earth Warrior* (1995). He is Associate Editor of the journal *Literature and Medicine,* has lectured widely on pain to medical audiences, and has held fellowships from the American Council of Learned Societies, the National Endowment for the Humanities, the National Science Foundation, and the Guggenheim Foundation.

Donald D. Price obtained a Ph.D. from the University of California at Davis in 1969 in the field of neurophysiology. After postdoctoral work at the U.C.L.A. Brain Research Institute, he held positions as physiologist and psychologist at the National Institutes for Health (Dental Institute); and as an Assistant (1971–1974), Associate (1980–1988), and full Professor (1988–present) in the Department of Anesthesiology, Medical College of Virginia. He is the author or coauthor of over 160 publications in the field of neural and psychological mechanisms of pain. He published a book on that subject in 1988, *Psychological and Neural Mechanisms of Pain* (Raven Press).

Arthur Shapiro earned his B.S.S. from the City College of New York in 1951 and his M.D. from the University of Chicago in 1955. He was a Clinical Professor of Psychiatry at the Mount Sinai School of Medicine in New York from 1977–1995. Arthur Shapiro is coauthor, with Elaine Shapiro, of *Gilles de la Tourette Syndrome* (Raven Press, 1978 first edition, 1988 second edition).

Elaine Shapiro received her B.A. from the City College of New York in 1953 and her Ph.D. from the University of Chicago in 1963. She has been an Assistant Clinical Professor of Psychiatry at Mount Sinai School of Medicine in New York since 1977. Elaine Shapiro is coauthor, with Arthur Shapiro, of *The Powerful Placebo* (Johns Hopkins University Press, 1997).

Howard Spiro is a leading gastroenterologist and the editor of the *Journal for Clinical Gastroenterology*. He began his training at Harvard University, Massachusetts General Hospital, and the Peter Bent Brigham Hospital in Boston. He is currently Professor of Medicine at Yale University School of Medicine, where he also directs the program for Humanities in Medicine. In addition, he is the author of *Doctors, Patients and Placebos*, published by Yale University Press in 1986, and is the editor of *Empathy and the Practice of Medicine: Beyond Pills and the Scalpel.*

Index

Acupuncture, 16–17, 28, 82
Addiction. *See* Drugs, active: addiction and withdrawal
Addiction model of placebo response, 130–132
Ader, Robert, 5, 6, 9, 84, 208, 225, 226, 227
Adherence to treatment. *See* Compliance
Administration of drugs and placebos, 19–20, 29, 97, 100, 112, 143; patient guesses about active vs. placebo treatment, 21, 31, 68, 151, 152, 227–228; prior, 31, 102, 120, 139, 141, 146, 147, 149, 150, 152; anxiety and, 105; chronic pain and, 111; placebo following active drug, 120, 146–147, 158; repeated, 172. *See also* Dosage(s)
Affect, associated, 56, 220, 221; affective dimension of pain, 133–134, 193, 235
Alcohol and placebo alcohol, 167, 169, 172–173, 175, 179, 196
Allocation of treatment. *See* Administration of drugs and placebos; Dosage(s)
Alternative medicine and treatment, 24, 27, 29, 44, 51
Analgesia: hypnotic, 30, 122–123, 133, 225; behavioral, 105, 111; conditioned, 106, 108, 109, 111–112, 174
Analgesia, placebo (general discussion), 4–5, 129–132; study and models of, 95–100, 104, 112–113, 117–132; associative learning and, 101–103, 104
Analgesics, 21, 25–26, 28, 38, 46, 94, 105. *See also* Drugs, active; Drugs, placebo; *specific or type of drugs*
Anesthesia, 190, 226, 227
Angiotensin, 86
Animal studies, 5–6, 226; fear, 65, 120, 219; conditioned response, 84, 141–142, 144–145, 152–153, 158, 160, 170, 189; neural, 96, 101; pain, 96, 102, 111, 112, 152–153; conditioned analgesia, 103–104, 109, 112, 152; disease models, 144, 154, 160, 227; taste aversion, 154–155; hope of survival, 221–222; sudden death syndrome, 221

Antianxiety drugs, 133
Antibodies, 142, 157
Antidepressants, 21, 63, 167, 194, 235
Antigen, 142, 157
Anxiety, 4, 30, 31, 45, 59, 180; pain and, 4, 104–105, 128, 133–134, 216; as factor in placebo effect, 25, 50, 128; panic disorder, 59, 63, 121, 174, 178; nocebos and, 61; placebo analgesia and, 104–105, 111–112, 117–118, 120, 127, 130, 218; reduction, 130, 133, 134, 175, 177; physicians and, 234–236. *See also* Stress
Approach goal, 130, 131, 132
Artifact(s), 2, 191; placebo effect as, 167–169, 180, 232, 243
Aspirin, 28, 40, 119, 122, 146
Asthma studies, 66–67
Atenolol, 149
Autonomy movement, 39, 44, 237–238, 239, 242
Aversion (defensive behavior), 96, 101, 178, 179; withdrawal reflex, 106, 112; taste aversion studies, 154–155. *See also* Threat, pain as
Avoidance goal, 130, 131, 132
Awareness, subjective, 93, 94. *See also* Cognition; Consciousness; Experience

Barrucand, D., 56, 57
Barsky, Arthur, 208
Beecher, Henry, 2, 3
Behavior, 87, 88; therapy, 26, 89; analgesia and, 105–106, 109, 111. *See also* Conditioning; Conditioning, classical
Belief, 30, 41, 188; in effectiveness of placebo, 27, 138, 139, 166, 175; physician's role in, 189; pain and, 188, 191, 192, 195; human health and, 200. *See also* Expectation(s); Faith; Hope
Benson, Herbert, 208, 212
Biochemical pathways/mediators, 2, 84, 85, 86, 87, 88, 213

Bioculturalism, 202; as factor in pain, 10, 188, 189, 190, 195, 201, 202; as factor in placebo effect, 196–197, 199–201

Biology, peripheral, 226, 227. *See also* Neurobiology

Biomedicine, 5, 40, 79, 81, 187, 192, 196, 233–235, 243–244, 248; models, 246

Blind testing. *See* Clinical studies: double-blind procedure

Bloodletting, 18

Brain, 2, 27, 245; emotions and, 86; activity, 93, 94, 95; conscious experience and, 93, 94; placebo analgesia and, 95, 108–111; circuitry, 96, 101, 104, 105–111, 112, 215, 218, 228, 235; stimulation studies, 109; models of, 245–246. *See also* Neuroscience *and related entries*

Brandt, Allan, 208

Brody, Howard, 9–10, 208, 229, 230, 241

Bruner, Jerome, 80, 229

Caffeine, 173

Cancer, 26, 42, 49, 50–51, 150, 179, 223

Cannon, Walter, 56, 65, 220

Causation theory, 29–30, 78

Chlorpromazine, 145, 170

Cimetidine, 41, 43

Classical conditioning. *See* Conditioning, classical

Clinical studies, 19, 27, 29–31; double-blind procedure, 1, 20–21, 22, 28, 40, 63, 96–97, 110, 238, 239; placebo control groups, 1, 20, 21–23, 28, 40–44, 63, 118, 138–139, 143, 147–150, 158, 175–176, 217; methodological difficulties, 8, 26, 28, 29, 67; single-blind procedure, 22; of surgery, 22, 28; of psychoanalysis, 23; replication requirement, 26, 27, 29, 168; FDA and, 27, 28; of drugs, 28, 40–44, 138–139, 140, 142, 156, 158, 187; randomized, 40, 41, 42–44, 47; criticism of, 42–44; outcome studies, 42; of nocebo effect, 66–67; sampling bias, 217

Clinical practice, 28, 39, 44, 50, 51, 78. *See also* Physician(s)

Cognition, 178, 233–234; as factor in placebo response, 83–84, 87, 189, 224; emotions and, 86; as factor in placebo analgesia, 121–123, 127–128

Compliance, 26, 41, 42, 167–169

Conditioned response. *See* Response: conditioned (CR)

Conditioning, 49, 225–229; as predictor of placebo response, 6, 9, 30, 84, 87, 119–121, 140–142; reinforcement schedules, 84, 143–144, 145, 150, 155, 156, 157–159, 174; fear and pain modulation and, 101; placebo analgesia and, 102, 119–121, 127, 173; analgesia response in humans, 106, 108, 117, 119, 124; models of learning and, 123; vs. expectation and desire, 124–125, 127, 147, 152, 166, 175; vs. experience, 126–127; role in pharmacotherapy, 140, 142–155, 159, 160; trials, 142, 145,

155, 159, 169, 173–174, 175; crossover studies of drug effects, 146–150, 152; sequence effects, 146; model of pharmacotherapy, 155–159; instrumental, 157, 158; models of stimulus substitution, 169–171; reversal of, 171; informational view of, 171–172, 174. *See also* Animal studies; Response

Conditioning, classical, 142, 158; placebo effects/response and, 6, 119, 121, 189; placebo analgesia and, 103, 104, 111–112, 117, 120, 122, 173; models, 120, 169–171, 173, 174–175; learning and expectation in, 123, 166, 226; vs. experience, 127; magnitude of placebo effect and, 127, 180; partial reinforcement effect and, 157; role of information in, 171–172, 174, 175

Consciousness/conscious mind, 10, 93, 94, 225–229

Consent. *See* Informed consent

Counterfeit placebos, 24

Couvade syndrome, 191

Crossover studies, 146–150, 152. *See also* Research and studies

Culturalist programs, 247

Culture of Pain, The (Morris), 192

Culture/cultural: sciences, 7–8, 10; environment and, 83; pain and, 190, 191–193, 195, 196; image of medicine, 196, 199; narrative, 196; mind and, 200–201; neurobiology and, 200, 233–234; symbols, 232. *See also* Sociocultural frameworks

Cyclophosphamide (CY), 5, 144, 154, 155, 226, 227

Death, 234; voodoo, 9, 56, 57, 59, 65–66, 71, 196, 220–222; adherence to treatment and, 42; expectations of, 56, 60, 221; fulfilled expectations of, 56, 60–61, 62, 65, 69; fear of, 59, 62, 65, 221; depression and, 60, 66; risk factors, 60–61; suicide, 64–65; timing of, 231–232. *See also* Survival

Definitions: placebo, 2, 12–13, 40, 44–45, 78–79, 187; placebo effect, 12, 78, 138, 139, 243–244; pain, 37, 38; disease, 45; illness, 45; nocebo, 56–59; expectation, 57; analgesic placebo response, 96; placebo analgesic effect, 96

Dehydration, 17–19, 65–66

Depression, 26, 211; symptoms, 18, 59, 66; treatment, 21, 25, 26, 167, 235; effect on physical illness, 26; deaths attributed to, 60, 66; placebo analgesia and, 130; expectancy and response in, 178–179, 180; pain and, 194

Desire for relief, 6, 84, 105, 117, 222, 223; as factor in placebo analgesia, 117–118, 125–127; /expectation model, 129–132; measurement of, 129

Deviance, 62–63

Diagnosis, 31, 53, 59, 62, 68, 213; of pain, 28; as placebo, 48, 194

Diazepam, 104, 111, 133

Digitalis (foxglove), 19, 39

Disease, 40, 43–46, 48, 187, 210, 216; place-bos and, 49, 50, 211, 216–218; nosological categories, 59, 69, 89; chronic, 60, 84; symptomatology, 64, 211–212; as object, 81; epidemic, 197, 198; vs. illness, 211–216, 226; natural course of, 216–218; social course of, 218. *See also* Animal studies: disease models; Illness/sickness

Dosage(s), 152; ineffective, 12, 28, 157; un-standardized, 19; in clinical tests, 21; in-creased, 21, 100, 156–157; -related effects, 102; -response relationship, 120, 153; cumu-lative, 143, 155–156, 158; maintenance lev-els, 160; decreased, 229

Dreams, 221

Drug companies, 192

Drugs, active, 20, 63, 119; new, 1, 14, 20–21, 27, 40–44, 158; prior experience with, 31, 102, 120, 139, 141, 146, 147, 149, 150, 152; cost of, 43, 159, 160; addiction and withdrawal, 53, 141, 142, 157; repeated ad-ministration (extinction), 120, 121, 141, 149, 157–158, 172, 173, 174–175; action of, 138, 139; treatment protocols, 139, 140, 151, 157; residual effects of, 147–148, 149–150; reinforcement schedules, 149, 155, 156; site of action, 151–152, 172; tolerance to, 151, 152; /placebo ratio, 155, 158; de-sign, 160; trials, 187. *See also* Analgesics; Clinical studies; Pharmacotherapy; Side ef-fects; *specific drugs and types of drugs*

Drugs, placebo, 30, 42, 167, 170, 172, 175; active, 13, 21, 28, 41–42, 120, 121, 138, 145; historical use of, 13–19; inactive or in-ert, 20, 28, 42, 44, 46, 79, 140, 142–143, 166; ineffective, 28. *See also* specific drugs and types of drugs

Eastwell, H. D., 65–66

Emergency situations and pain, 119, 190, 220

Emotions, 71, 83, 128, 129; placebo response and, 86, 87, 130; expectation and, 130; pain and, 194. *See also* Mental states and disorders

End organs. *See* Target organ response

Endorphins, 4–5, 48, 49, 50, 175, 177, 188, 189

Engel, George L., 39, 194, 230

Environment/context, 235; social, 68–69, 70, 83, 247; factors in placebo analgesia, 95, 103, 112, 117, 118–119, 121, 152. *See also* Stimuli: environmental

Ephedrine, 16

Escape response (fight or flight), 220

Ethics and ethical issues, 1, 39, 42–43; pla-cebo as deception of patient, 39, 78, 82, 236–242; in studying nocebo effect, 66, 67; in neuroscientific experimentation, 101; in-formed consent, 125, 158, 237, 238–239; physicians and, 234–242

Ethnic groups, 192, 193

Euphoria, 132

Expectation(s), 9, 27, 44, 49–50, 117, 123, 222, 223, 225; positive, 30, 57; affective states and, 56, 59; cultural environment and, 56, 69–70; of death, 56, 60–61, 62, 65, 69, 221; negative, 56–57, 59, 61, 62, 67, 69, 71; types of, 57–58; worldview and, 60–61; based on prior experience, 67, 120–121, 123, 125, 226; behavioral and social, 70–71; placebo stimuli and, 84, 171, 172, 174, 180; placebo analgesia and, 118, 122, 123–125, 128; vs. conditioning, 124–125, 147, 152, 171; manipulation, 124–125, 126, 173; measures of, 124, 125, 129; im-plicit, 126–127; emotions and, 130; re-sponse, 166, 172; theory, 171–175; subjective response and, 175–180; unmedi-ated effects of, 177–179; desire and, 223, 224. *See also* Belief; Faith; Hope

Experience: common, 93, 126; subjective, 93, 94, 95, 101, 178–179, 224; sensory, 102; of pain, 122, 190–191, 192, 211; as factor in placebo effect, 126–127, 134; symbolic forms of, 230–231

Extinction. *See* Drugs, active: repeated admini-stration

Extinction test, 121

Fads in healing, 24

Faith, 175, 222; and healing, 7, 10, 24, 50, 60, 196, 234; in power of placebos, 24–25, 128; in technology, 27; role of, 41, 42, 48–49, 146, 222; as factor in placebo analgesia, 30, 117–118, 122, 127, 128, 176, 177; re-ligious behavior, 223–224. *See also* Belief; Expectation(s); Hope

Family practice model, 240–241

FDA (Food and Drug Administration), 27, 28, 43

Fear: to die of, 10, 50; as factor in placebo ef-fect, 25, 104–105, 111–112, 117–118, 120, 219–220; of death, 59, 62, 65, 221; condi-tioned, 101, 103–104, 120; placebo analgesia and, 104–105; of drugs, 177; ex-pectation and, 178; pain and, 194, 220

Fields, Howard, 4, 9, 84, 208, 217, 219, 226

Fraud/quackery, 24, 29, 77, 78, 189, 235, 236, 238. *See also* Ethics and ethical issues

Functional imaging methods (MRI, PET), 95, 112, 113, 216

Galen, 13, 14, 17, 42, 187

Gastroenterology and use of endoscopy, 37, 39, 41, 211, 238, 240

Gate Control Theory of Pain, 245

Genetics, 139, 200, 212

Gold, H., 20

Guessing about placebo vs. drugs, 21, 31, 68, 151, 152, 227–228

Hahn, Robert A., 6, 9

Harrington, Anne, 208

Harvard Medical School, 234, 237

Harvard Mind, Brain, Behavior Interfaculty In-itiative, 8, 10

Healing: symbolic, 7, 10, 44; herbal remedies, 14–19, 39, 197, 198; natural course of, 40,

43, 216–218; ceremonies, 44, 197–198, 199; self-, 47, 240; faith, 50, 196; stimuli, 80–85; theories of, 233

Heart disease, 29; angina pectoris, 20, 22, 48, 188; attacks and strokes, 26, 28, 42, 57–58; ischemic, 60, 61; fear of, 61; sudden cardiac death, 221

Herbal medicine, 14–19, 39, 197, 198

History of placebos and placebo effects, 18–19, 31, 40, 199–200; in prescientific medicine, 13–19; in scientific medicine, 19–27, 39

Holistic treatments, 24, 25, 52–53

Homeopathy, 49, 199

Homeostasis, 154, 156

Hope, 176, 177, 222; role in placebo analgesia and effect, 18, 30, 40, 117–118, 128, 175, 180; of survival, 221–222; meaning construction and, 223–224; pain and, 223. *See also* Belief; Expectation(s); Faith

Hopelessness, 26, 58, 59, 176, 177, 222

Hugdahl, Kenneth, 208

Hyman, Steven, 244, 208–209

Hyperalgesia, 110, 111

Hypertension, 46, 149, 188, 212

Hypnosis/hypnotic analgesia, 30, 122–123, 133, 225

Hypochondriasis, 59, 61

Hypotensive drug effects, 152

Hysteria, 45, 63–64

Identity, 70

Identification with other victims, 71

Illness/sickness, 40, 45–46, 48, 218; "holiday," 10, 231; expectations of, 56, 59, 69; psychogenic, 63–64; sociogenic, 63–65, 68, 70; nocebo effect and, 65–67, 69; repertoire, 69; meaningful explanations of, 81, 82, 87; vs. disease, 211–216, 226. *See also* Disease

Imagery, 122, 126

Imaging methods, 95, 112, 113, 216

Immediate relations/links, 178, 179

Immune system, 5, 9, 24, 26–27, 154; pathways and placebo effects, 84, 85, 227; response, 134, 142, 144, 179

Immunosuppresive therapy, 144, 145, 155, 156

Indomethacin, 146

Information/knowledge, 122, 123, 134, 235, 240; classical conditioning and, 171–172, 174, 175; verbal, 172, 173–174; as factor in placebo effect, 176. *See also* Learning

Informed consent, 125, 158, 237, 238–239

Intention vs. volition, 178

Intensions (voluntary response), 166

International Association for the Study of Pain (IASP), 190, 192, 195

Interpersonal relations. *See* Patient: /physician relationship

Intuition, 38–39

Jensen, Michael, 209

Kaufman, Gordon, 209, 229

Kennedy, W. P., 56, 57

Kirsch, Irving, 6, 9, 84, 121, 209, 224

Kissel, P., 56, 57

Kleinman, Arthur, 6, 83, 209, 231, 235

Knowledge. *See* Information/knowledge; Learning

Kosslyn, Stephen, 209, 232

Labeling theory, 62–63, 82

Language, 190, 210, 238, 245

Learning, 101–103, 169; associative, 6, 101–103, 104; role in placebo analgesia, 101–103, 104, 119–121, 122; prior, 102, 226, 227; models, 123; conditioned response and, 141–142, 171; as mechanism, 154; state-dependent, 158; placebo effect and, 159; pain and, 189–190, 195

Leeching, 18

Levine, J. D., 100, 110, 111

Lithium chloride, 154

MacArthur Research Network on Mind-Body Interactions, 8

Magic, spirituality, and supernatural belief systems, 38, 39, 51, 53, 66, 82, 198–200. *See also* Shamans; Voodoo death

Magnetic resonance imaging (MRI), 112

Magnitude: of placebo effect, 118, 119, 127, 152, 153, 174, 180. *See also* Pain: severity

Malpractice issues, 241

Managed care, 241

Manipulation: placebo, 101, 117, 118, 120, 122, 126, 133, 134; expectancy, 124–125, 126, 130, 173; of conditioning, 125, 130; of motivation, 126; experimental, 129; desire and, 130; cognitive, 133. *See also* Conditioning; Stimuli: conditioned (CS)

Mass hysteria, 63–64

Mauss, Marcel, 65

Meaning(s), 122; -making, 9–10, 223–224, 229–231; pain and, 190, 191–192, 194; hope and, 223–224

Meaning model of placebo action, 9–10, 79–80, 87–89, 188, 189; narration in, 9, 80–81, 84; healing stimuli, 80–85; role of society and culture, 82–83; neurobiology of meaning, 85–87

Measurement: estimates of placebo effect, 21; of improvement, 49; of expectations, 124, 125, 129. *See also* Scaling procedures

Mechanisms, 8, 78, 187, 202; physiological, 8, 59, 71; psychological, 9; placebo, 22, 94, 95, 177, 178; unexplained functioning of, 40, 49–51, 138, 177, 188, 197, 243; neural, 95–96, 100–101, 102, 104, 105, 112, 113; brain, 245

Medical institutions, 138, 234

Medical practice, 53, 93; science and, 8, 38, 39, 43, 51, 52

Medical students' disease (MSD), 61

Medicine, 27, 77; primitive/herbal, 13–19, 39, 196–200; homeopathic, 49, 199; primary care, 84

Memory, 95, 101, 123, 124, 129

Mental states and disorders, 25, 26, 50; physical manifestation of, 18, 26, 50, 85, 93, 94; therapies for, 23; placebo effects and, 27; psychological profiles, 42; expectations and, 59, 61; social origins of, 62–63; physiology and, 85. *See also* Emotions
Migraine headaches, 97–98
Milk, 48
Mind-body dualism, 37, 39, 47, 50, 51, 187, 220; use of placebos and, 26, 27, 78, 85, 233; as common experience, 93–94; therapies, 212
Morphine, 4, 21, 94, 100, 105, 107, 118, 119, 141, 170; placebo, 122, 141, 170; in animal studies, 152
Morris, David B., 10
Motivation, 30, 49, 123, 223, 218–220
Multiplicative model of placebo response, 129–130, 133
Multiplicity, 89

Naloxone, 4, 88, 104, 109, 110–111, 112, 133, 168, 177
Naming. *See* Labeling theory
Narratives/storytelling, 9, 10, 80–81, 84, 229–233, 235, 244, 247. *See also* Patient(s): listening to
Native American folk medicine, 197–199, 200
Near-death experiences, 221
Nervous system, central, 87, 94, 95, 96, 100, 105, 109, 111, 112, 187, 200, 215; diseases of, 28; pathways and connections, 37–38, 79, 80, 84, 85, 88, 95, 96, 105, 215; mechanisms of, 94–96, 100–101, 102, 104, 105, 112, 113, 218–220; neural hypothesis of placebo analgesia, 100–101, 108–111
Neuroanatomy, 80, 87, 88, 218
Neurobiology, 4, 88, 101, 189, 191, 192, 235, 247; of meaning, 85–87; neural representations, 94–95; placebo mechanisms and, 95, 189, 196, 200; cultural effects and, 200, 233–234; model of placebo effects, 244–245, 248
Neurochemistry, 88
Neuroimmunology, 50–51
Neuropeptides, 88, 89, 196
Neurophysiology, 9, 10, 88
Neuroscience, 4, 79, 248; cognitive, 233–234, 246
Neurotransmitters, 96, 104, 109, 112, 190, 195, 219
Nocebo(s)/nocebo effect, 9, 80, 98; voodoo death, 9, 56, 57, 59, 65–66, 71, 196, 220–222; cultural environment and, 56, 58, 68, 69–70, 71, 196, 197, 199, 200; working definition of, 56–59; pathological outcomes and, 57, 58, 59–60, 67, 68; as negative placebo, 57; deliberate vs. unintended, 58, 59, 71; evidence of, 59–67, 71; risk factors for, 60–61, 68, 69, 70, 71; social environment and, 64–65, 67, 68–69, 70, 71; study of, 66–69; behavioral model, 71
Nociception, 133, 190, 192. *See also* Pain
Nonplacebos, 19, 20, 31

Nonspecific response and treatments, 1–2, 12, 17, 23, 26, 42, 61, 62, 139, 176
Nosology, 59, 69, 89
No treatment groups, 17, 97, 98, 100, 118, 144, 147, 148–149, 150, 158. *See also* Clinical studies: placebo control groups; Pain: absence of treatment for

Oepen, Godehard, 188, 209
Opioid(s), 4, 109, 218; endogenous, 4, 5, 9, 25–26, 96, 105, 106, 109–110, 111–112, 177, 200, 219; antagonists, 88, 104, 106, 109–110, 177; -mediated analgesic response, 104; peptides, 105, 109; -mediated pain-modulating circuitry, 108–111, 112; exogenous, 109
Opium, 4, 14

Pain, 4, 22, 49, 50–51, 96, 242; psychological, 3, 28, 190, 193–195, 209–210; increase in, 4, 98, 109, 110; -modulating brain circuits, 9, 95, 96, 101, 105–111, 112–113, 189; biocultural approach to, 10, 188, 189, 190, 195, 201, 202; as punishment, 18, 38, 194; effectiveness of placebos on, 37–38, 41, 49, 53, 94–95, 97, 98; existential, 37, 38, 211; acute, 37–38, 45, 102, 109, 111, 118, 128, 189, 191, 209; chronic, 37, 38, 45, 189, 194, 210; perception and experience of, 40, 119, 122, 133–134, 139, 190–192, 194, 209–210, 218; nonspecific, 61, 62; reduction, 94, 100, 102–103, 117; environmental context for, 95, 103, 112, 117, 118–119; subjective, 96, 109; absence of treatment for, 97, 98–99, 100, 110, 118; duration (time course), 97, 98–99, 112, 120, 128; natural history of, 97, 98, 100, 110, 118, 119, 216; severity (magnitude), 97, 98, 99, 100, 112, 118–119, 128, 133, 193, 195; variable dimensions of, 97, 117, 118, 119, 122–123, 132–133, 193; clinical, 104, 110, 118, 128, 176; experimental, 104, 110, 118, 128, 133, 141, 153; transmission, 105–108, 192; ischemic, 110, 118; in emergency situations, 119, 190, 220; measurement, 132–134; affective dimensions of, 133–134, 193, 235; tolerance, 133, 190; physiological, 134, 218–219; beliefs, 188, 191, 192, 195; learning and, 189–190, 195; role of mind in, 192, 194; management, 195; medical model of, 195, 202; hope and, 223
Pancreas, 14–15
Pathophysiological processes, 134
Patient(s), 48–49, 81, 138; credulity of, 3, 25, 30; /physician relationship, 3, 9, 30, 39–40, 44–49, 51–53, 82–83, 90, 167–169, 177, 230, 231, 235, 239–240, 242, 244; profile as factor in outcomes, 3, 42, 50, 59–61; positive placebo reactors, 21, 22, 29–31, 42, 49, 50, 79–81, 97, 139, 147, 188, 217; autonomy of, 39, 44, 237–238, 239, 242; listening to, 39, 40, 47, 51, 52, 88, 247;

control over pain, 47, 195; social role of, 70, 71; as therapeutic agent, 90, 134
Pavlov conditioning. *See* Conditioning, classical
Penicillin, 17
Peptide receptors, 85–86, 87. *See also* Neuropeptides
Perceptual bias, 167–169
Performance inhibition, 172
Pert, Candace, 85, 86–87
Pharmacology, 112, 140. *See also* Drugs, active
Pharmacotherapy, 138, 159–160; role of conditioning in, 140, 142–155, 159, 160; conditioning model of, 155–159. *See also* Drugs, active
Physician(s): ethical considerations and skepticism about use of placebos, 1, 3, 38–40, 44, 46–47, 50, 53, 234–242; as therapeutic agent for placebo effect, 3, 9, 15, 77–78, 84, 90, 219, 225; loyalty and commitment to patients, 51–52, 54, 79, 80, 236, 240, 241–242; role of, 79, 81–83, 219; specialists, 214–215, 239. *See also* Patient(s): /physician relationship
Physiology, 4, 50, 85, 89, 215, 224; placebos and, 2, 5–6, 27, 44, 49, 127, 159, 168–169, 179–180, 212; of pain, 134, 218–219; conditioning and, 141–142, 153–154, 156; mechanisms of, 179–180
Placebo effect (general discussion), 18–19, 24–27, 29–30, 67–68, 156, 199–200; multiple, 133; duration of, 152, 174; models of, 153, 226
Placebo reactors. *See* Patient(s): positive placebo reactors
Positron emission tomography (PET), 95, 112, 216
Price, Donald, 9, 84, 209
Prior experience as factor in placebo response, 31, 139, 227–228; administration of drugs, 31, 102, 120, 139, 141, 146, 147, 149, 150, 152; expectations, 67, 120–121, 123, 125, 226; treatment or therapy, 117, 122, 128, 146
Psychiatry, 25, 29, 30, 51, 158, 171, 234–235
Psychoanalysis, 22–23, 230
Psychobiology, 139
Psychoimmunology, 26–27
Psychology/psychological functions, 2–3, 9, 201; pain and, 3, 28, 192, 193–195; placebo effects and, 12, 26, 27; in placebo analgesia, 117–118, 132; mediators as, 177–178, 180
Psychoneuroimmunology, 9
Psychopathology, 62
Psychopharmacology, 235
Psychophysiology, 12
Psychosomatic functioning, 50, 52, 85, 88, 223
Psychotherapy, 18, 23, 158, 229–231, 235; placebo effects in, 22–24, 25, 29; controlled studies of, 28, 31; narrative in, 232

Quackery. *See* Fraud/quackery

Randomized clinical trials (RCTs). *See* Clinical studies
Reductionist models, 88, 243–244, 245, 246
Reinforcement effect. *See* Conditioning
Relapse rates, 149, 152
Religion, 18, 223–224. *See also* Faith
Remedies, nonmedical, 13–19
REM sleep, 221
Replacement therapy, 159. *See also* Pharmacotherapy
Research and study, 10, 28, 40, 90, 125, 187–188; literature on, 2–7; interdisciplinary and multidisciplinary, 8, 90, 245; drug, 28, 40–44, 138–139, 142, 146–151; placebo effect, 30–31, 159, 234, 245; agendas, 78, 79–80, 83, 86–89; methods, 79, 84–85; mechanistic approaches, 83, 138; future, 88, 242–248; design, 138, 159, 160, 238; placebo manipulation, 117, 134; placebo analgesia, 123–124; pain, 133–134, 192, 193–194; psychopharmacology, 142, 155–159; pharmacotherapy, 144–146, 160; grants, 192, 238; cross-cultural, 192–193; neurobiology, 196; psychotherapy, 229–231; balanced placebo design, 238–239; ethics and, 238. *See also* Clinical studies; Conditioning: trials
Response: nonspecific, 1–2, 26; conditioned (CR), 47, 120, 121, 151, 153, 154, 160, 169–170, 172, 173, 174, 180, 225; unconditioned (UR or UCR), 120, 122, 140, 151, 169, 171–173; compensatory, 151–154, 171, 172, 175; pharmacologic, 153–155; pharmacotherapeutic, 153–155; expectancy, 166, 173, 174, 175–180; intention and, 178. *See also* Conditioning
Rituals and ceremonies of healing, 53, 88, 196, 198, 247
Rose, Robert, 209, 212

Saccharin/sugar pills, 1, 5, 12, 13, 46, 57, 144, 226
Scaling procedures (visual analog scales and line production), 84, 125, 129, 130, 132
Scarry, Elaine, 38, 209, 242, 247
Schizophrenia, 42, 145, 146, 149, 152, 228
Science, 7, 8, 38–39, 43, 51, 52, 82, 187
Self: -scrutiny, 59, 61, 96; -healing, 90, 196–197; -reporting, 96, 126, 168, 169; -limiting pain, 98; -confirming response expectancies, 174, 180
Sexual abuse, childhood, 194
Sexual arousal, male, 172, 176, 179
Shamans, 196, 197–198, 199, 234, 235, 236. *See also* Magic, spirituality, and supernatural belief systems
Shapiro, Arthur, 3, 8, 44, 200
Shapiro, Elaine, 8
Side effects, 228, 229: of drugs, 21, 28, 30–31, 150–151, 156; placebo-induced, 30–31, 44, 57, 176–177; nocebo-induced, 57, 58; of culture, 71; conditioned, 151; magnitude of, 157
Sleep, 190, 221

Sociocultural frameworks, 7, 8, 44, 45, 81, 88, 233, 239, 247
Socioeconomic frameworks, 241
Sociosemantic transformations, 232–233
Somatic illness, 4
Somatoform disorders, 59, 194
Sorcery. *See* Magic, spirituality and supernatural belief systems; Voodoo death
Specificity of placebo effects, 176–177, 180, 225
Spinal cord. *See* Brain: circuitry
Spiro, Howard, 8–9, 209, 236, 238, 247
Spontaneous remission, 22, 119, 167, 168, 175, 216
Stimulants, 167, 169, 175, 176, 179
Stimuli: conditioned (CS), 6, 119, 120, 121, 140–144, 149, 150, 152–154, 157, 159, 169, 226; placebo, 29, 30, 78, 81, 84, 87, 89, 90, 101, 143; meaningful, 80–85, 87, 88; environmental, 88, 101–102, 103, 112, 143, 149; social, 88; behavioral, 89; psychosocial, 89; sensory, 95, 102, 118, 141, 152, 154; pain and, 96, 102, 124, 173, 174, 177, 190–191, 218; noxious, 103, 106, 109, 112, 190, 218; neutral, 119, 120, 141, 153, 154, 159; UCS/CS association, 119, 120, 122, 127, 140, 144–145, 147, 148, 157, 158, 171, 174, 180; unconditioned (UCS or US), 119, 122, 123, 140, 150, 151, 153–154, 157, 159, 169–170, 172, 174, 175, 227; nociceptive, 133, 190, 192; antigenic, 142, 157; expectation and, 166; substitution models, 169–171, 172, 173, 175; emotional, 216; prior exposure to, 227–228
Stone, Alan, 209, 223
Storytelling. *See* Narratives/storytelling
Stress, 50, 51, 52, 64, 111, 112, 212, 221; pain and, 100, 104, 118. *See also* Anxiety
Sudden cardiac death, 221
Suicide, 64–65
Sullivan, Lawrence, 232, 245
Supernatural. *See* Magic, spirituality and supernatural belief systems
Surgery, 22, 27–29, 111
Survival, 26, 31, 49, 62, 197
Symbols/symbolism, 3, 7, 10, 44, 45, 53, 102, 231–232
Symptomatology, 64, 211–212
Symptoms, 69; of depression, 18, 59, 66; variations in, 22, 30; stress and, 51; control over, 79, 80, 82–83; sociogenic, 63–64; relief from, 80, 89–90, 119; -free periods, 158

Target organ response, 80, 85, 88, 151, 156, 157
Taste aversion, 154–155
Technology, 27, 213–214
Testing. *See* Clinical studies; Conditioning: trials
Therapeutic effect of placebos, 12, 24–25, 42, 43–44, 46, 142
Therapeutic relationship, 175–176, 177
Thoits, P. A., 70
Threat, 118, 119, 128, 220. *See also* Fear
Time: as factor in healing, 40, 43, 216–218; consciousness of, 229, 230, 232, 233. *See also* Pain: duration (time course)
Tranquilizers: active, 121, 146, 152, 153, 170, 171, 176; placebo, 145, 167, 169, 170–171, 172, 175, 176, 179
Treatment/therapies: nonspecific, 23, 26; medical, 27–28, 134; placebos as, 44–49; protocols, 84, 139, 140, 151, 157; manipulation, 97; prior, 117, 122, 128, 146; adherence to, 212. *See also* No treatment groups
Trust, 175, 177, 239–240
Types of placebos: sugar, saccharin, 1, 5, 12, 13, 46, 57, 144, 226; inert, 12, 28; surgery, 22, 27, 48; pill forms, 44, 48, 122, 140, 170, 176, 189; procedure forms, 44, 48; impure vs. pure, 47–48; injections, 48, 117, 122, 140, 170, 176, 189

Ulcers, 41, 43, 52–53, 188, 211
Unconscious processes, 83

Variation: of symptoms, 22, 30; in placebo effects, 43, 130, 235. *See also* Pain: variable dimensions of
Visual analog scales. *See* Scaling procedures
Vitamins and nutrition, 24, 25, 27–28
Voodoo death, 9, 56, 57, 59, 65–66, 71, 196, 220–222

Wash out periods. *See* Clinical studies: placebo control groups; No treatment groups
Wickramasekera, I., 119–120
Will to live, 10. *See also* Survival
Wolf, Stewart, 6, 168
Words as placebos, 53–54, 71. *See also* Narratives/storytelling; Patient(s): listening to

Yale Medical School, 234